CRAZY BUSY
BEAUTIFUL

Also by Carmindy

The 5-Minute Face

Get Positively Beautiful

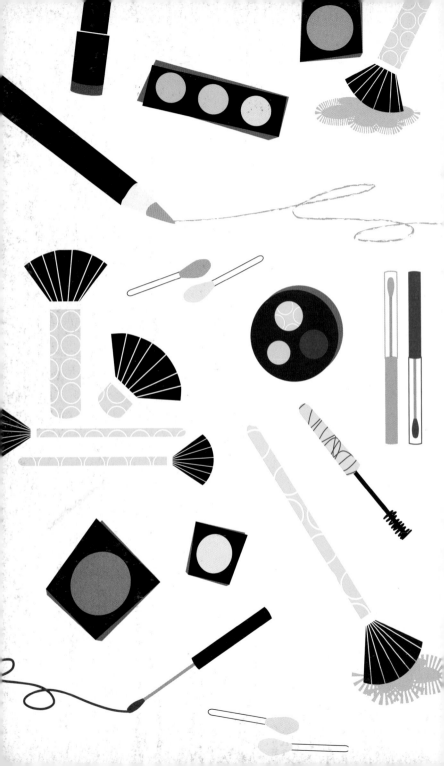

CRAZY BUSY
BEAUTIFUL

Beauty Secrets for
Getting Gorgeous Fast

CARMINDY

Illustrations by Amy Saidens

harperstudio
An Imprint of HarperCollins*Publishers*

HarperCollins books may be purchased for educational, business, or sales promotional use. For information please write: Special Markets Department, HarperCollins Publishers, 10 East 53rd Street, New York, NY 10022.

For more information about this book or other books from HarperStudio, visit www .theharperstudio.com.

FIRST EDITION

Library of Congress Cataloging-in-Publication Data
Carmindy.
   Crazy busy beautiful : beauty secrets for getting gorgeous fast / by Carmindy.—1st ed.
     p. cm.
  ISBN 978-0-06-185202-2 (pbk.)
1.   Beauty, Personal.   I. Title.
  RA778.C21673 2010
  646.7'2—dc22

                                 2009043361

10 11 12 13 14   OV/RRD   10 9 8 7 6 5 4 3 2 1

To my girlfriends.

Through busy times, frustratingly slow points,
crazy days, and even nuttier nights, you've filled
my life with beauty, care, and laughter.

I love you all to bits!

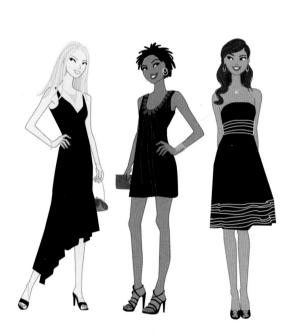

Contents

CRAZY BUSY
BEAUTIFUL

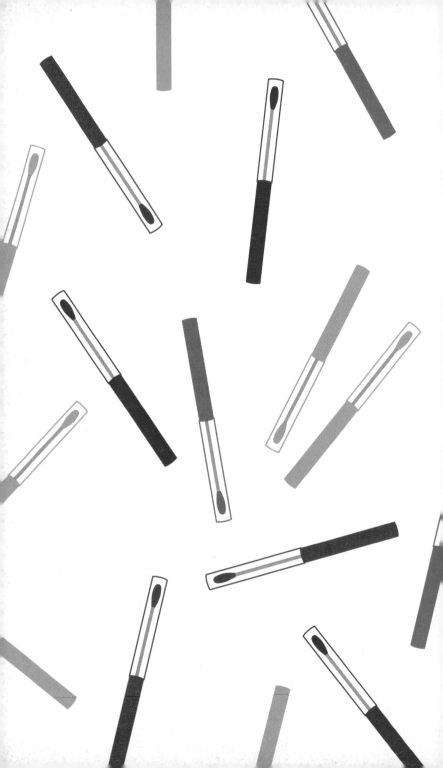

Tip
Numero
Uno

Trust your girlfriends.

We're all leading such crazy busy lives. Where can you turn for rock-solid advice? To the women you trust. Friends, teachers, grandmothers, mothers, aunties, sisters, and—when it comes to beauty—me.

I consider each of you to be one of my girlfriends. What you think, how you feel, and what you need and want to learn all guide me every day.

Sharing beauty secrets is just one way we women help each other make our crazy busy lives more beautiful. It's fun passing along tips! It's fun pawing through our pals' makeup bags and figuring out what brings out our best! And it's fun celebrating our unique gifts—united in loveliness!

This book compiles all the beauty secrets I have learned as a makeup artist. But I know enough to know I don't know everything. So I asked fans, friends, and family to share theirs. From the budget-savvy to the downright wacky, ladies across the globe graciously contributed their wisdom to help you shine.

Your end of the deal? To share what you learn with the women you love. Getting gorgeous is a team sport. So let's get busy cheering each other on!

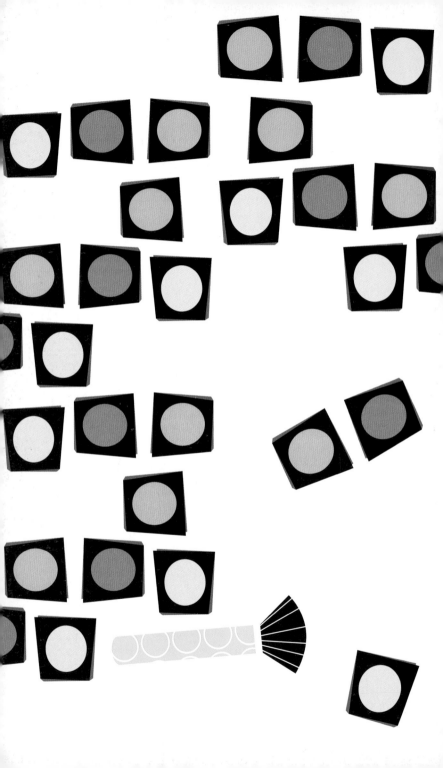

Start *with* Skin Care

Skin tells all. It reflects your health, indicates your stress-o-meter, and shows whether you've made prevention part of your beauty routine.

Even if you haven't been most excellent to your epidermis, fear not. It's never too late (or too soon) to step up your skin-care routine and reap the gorgeous rewards.

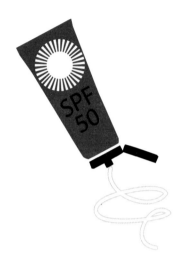

Wear sunscreen every single day. Nothing prevents wrinkles, aging, and spots like a big slather of SPF 30 or higher. Clouds. Rain. Snow. Sun. No matter what, wear it!

✳ The best sunscreens contain ingredients like zinc or titanium dioxide. These provide your skin with a stronger barrier of protection. They may take a bit longer to blend in, but they work very well when applied early and often.

✳ It is a myth that any protection over SPF 15 is a waste. You need a 30 or higher SPF to stay protected. And don't be stingy with sunscreen: you need a full coating for full-power protection.

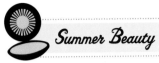
Summer Beauty

Despite the name, waterproof sunscreen still needs to be reapplied after you get out of the water. Even if you're not taking a dip, you should still reapply every two hours.

✳ If sunscreen stings your eyes, switch to a formula made for the eye area. In a pinch, apply a lip balm with a high SPF around your eyes.

✳ If you go to the beach and notice a million more freckles emerging by day's end, you are not protecting yourself enough. Use the highest SPF possible, wear a hat, and sit under an umbrella.

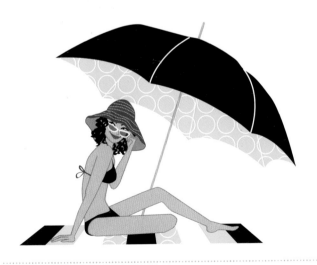

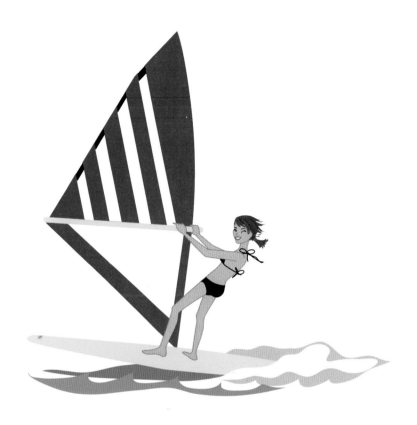

✳ When using a high-SPF sunscreen, always apply it after your moisturizer and let it soak in before applying makeup.

✳ If your high-SPF sunscreen leaves a noticeable white cast on your face, mix in a bit of foundation before your application to create an even, natural look.

✳ Not sure how to reapply sunscreen over your makeup without messing it up? Simply spritz on a spray sunscreen over your face—no blending necessary.

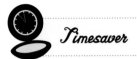

Timesaver

Choose a moisturizer with SPF for a quick one-two punch. It simultaneously protects your skin and keeps it supple.

The Nasties

SUNBURNS

Did you commit the biggest beauty sin—frying your face?! Be glad I'm not there to see it; sunburns burn me up! Now, after promising yourself never to let this happen again, take some aspirin or ibuprofen to reduce the pain and inflammation. Then moisturize like crazy with aloe—based moisturizers. Before going out, slather on sunscreen and put on a face—shading hat.

To cover up sunburn, tap—don't rub— liquid foundation onto the skin, using a non—latex sponge. Dust on a yellow—based powder to reduce redness.

Since you've charred your skin red, avoid wearing blush. Choose tawny or neutral lip colors (without a hint of red or pink) to tone down the red—alert effect.

✳ Wash your face at night. You don't have to cleanse again in the morning unless you get really oily. Over-washing can dry out your skin.

✳ Never, ever sleep in your makeup! No matter how tired you are, always remove your makeup and apply mois-turizer before going to bed. You'll thank me in the morning.

✳ For dry skin, choose creamy cleansers and cream moisturizers.

✳ For oily skin, go for gel cleansers and oil-free mois-turizing lotions.

✳ If you're a soap-and-water girl, never use regular body soap on your face. Choose pH-balanced facial soaps suited to your skin type.

✳ Using a terry-cloth washcloth to wash your face can help slough off dead skin cells.

✳ If you are prone to ruddiness, never use really hot water. It can irritate capillaries and cause further redden-ing.

* Mix a small amount of baking soda with a drop of liquid facial cleanser for lighter, brighter-looking skin without bleaching.

* Swipe a cotton ball dipped in mineral oil across stubborn makeup. It will melt off.

* To remove eye makeup, use soft cotton squares dipped in makeup remover and wipe gently. Avoid using toilet paper: it's too abrasive.

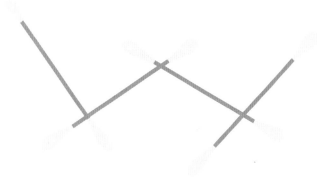

* Dip a Q-tip into makeup remover and sweep across the lash line to remove waterproof eyeliner.

* Baby wipes are handy for removing stubborn eye makeup. Carry a couple of individually wrapped baby wipes in case you end up on a pal's sofa at four A.M.

* If you're stuck without your usual cleanup gear, clear lip gloss can be used as an eye makeup remover.

＊ Exfoliate your face at least a few times a week. A good scrub eliminates dry flakes, sebum, oils, and any other nasty things that keep your skin from being supersmooth.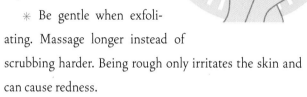

＊ Be gentle when exfoliating. Massage longer instead of scrubbing harder. Being rough only irritates the skin and can cause redness.

＊ Plain white sugar is hands-down the best exfoliant around. In the shower, simply lather up your face and body with your regular cleanser and then scrub about a handful of sugar over your skin, using circular motions. Rinse away remaining crystals. You'll be glowingly sweet.

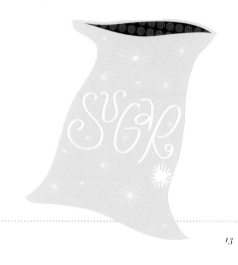

※ Avoid alcohol-based toners. They just strip your skin of its natural oils. If you like to tone, choose herbal toners like rosewater.

 Moneysaver

Apple cider vinegar makes a great—if a bit stinky—natural toner. Fill your sink with cool water and add about a cup of the stuff. Splash your face multiple times; rinse with plain cold water.

※ Splash your face with cold water before applying your moisturizer, to help tighten up the skin.

※ To see if a moisturizer is rich enough for you, do the tight test. Apply it and wait for a few minutes. If your skin still feels tight, you need to step up to a heavier, richer formula.

※ Don't skip moisturizer if you have oily skin. You may be making it oilier by skipping, as your glands may be overproducing oil to protect your skin. Reduce their workload! Smooth on a little oil-free moisturizer every morning.

※ Always carry a sample size of your moisturizer in your purse. If you get dry, you can easily reapply throughout the day.

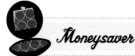

Moneysaver

Olive oil serves as a good natural moisturizer for super-dry skin.

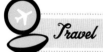

Travel

Headed for the airport? Skip the makeup and reapply moisturizer throughout the flight to keep your skin hydrated.

✳ If you're going to splurge on a skin product, put your big bucks down for an eye cream that's packed with age-fighting ingredients. The newest formulas can create a visible difference. I've seen it on my own peepers.

✳ Regular moisturizer doubles just fine as an eye cream if you don't want to blow the extra dough.

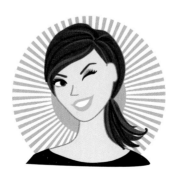

* Make your expensive face cream last longer by applying it only where you need it most. Use bargain moisturizer elsewhere.

* For a quick-n-easy eye cream, tap a rich lip salve around the crow's-feet area of the eyes.

* Always use your ring finger—the weakest digit—to apply eye cream. It will keep you from pulling or tugging the delicate skin around your eyes.

* Applying rich natural oils at night can really help quench parched, thirsty skin. Try neroli oil, argan oil, or sweet almond oil. Be sure to buy these from a reputable source. Steer clear if you're prone to breakouts.

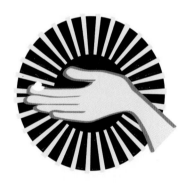

✳ Keep your creams stashed in the refrigerator during the summer for a cool, refreshing twist to your skincare regimen.

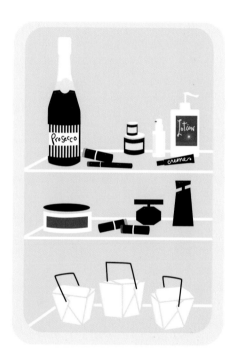

✳ The T-zone runs across your forehead, down the nose, and onto the chin. Oil glands cluster in the T-zone, so it tends to get shinier faster. Some shine looks youthful. But to reduce excessive oiliness, apply a mattifying gel after your moisturizer.

The Nasties

ZITS

If you feel a pimple coming on, hold an ice cube on the area to minimize swelling. Then dab a little clay mask on the spot and leave it on overnight.

Take the red out of a pimple by dabbing it with chilled Visine using a clean Q—tip. (I always keep my Visine in the fridge for this. Plus, if I need it for red eyes, it's more soothing when it's cold.)

A touch of lemon juice will dry out a zit in a flash.

To dry out a deep zit overnight, try applying a paste made out of baking soda and a little water.

Salicylic acid gel is the best thing to clear up pimples. After washing your face, apply this serum to the problem area. You should see a speedy improvement.

A clay mask can help dry up acne. The clay's drawing properties can also reduce pimples that haven't yet surfaced.

Drugstore products can't effectively treat

severe acne. Save your face from potential scarring: see a dermatologist about potent, prescription—only treatments like Retin—A.

Never cover breakouts with heavy foundation. Choose a light, oil—free liquid makeup or airbrush spray makeup and then spot—conceal where you need it.

Cover a pimple and help get rid of it at the same time. Look for concealers that contain zit—zapping ingredients—like salicylic acid.

If a cheek pimple is still visible through your blush, dab on a little concealer and powder. Then, using a Q—tip, lightly dab a mixture of blush and face powder onto the spot for an even look.

If you have a zit that has dried up and is a bit flaky, just spot—conceal. Go easy on the powder or skip it altogether so as not to accentuate the dryness.

Got a giant North Star zit that concealer just won't camouflage? First, remember it's a zit, not a death sentence. Don't give a pustule the power to ruin your day! Redirect your feature focus. Sweep on a bright bold lipstick to draw attention to your beaming smile!

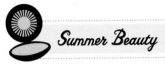

Summer Beauty

If you get super-shiny in the hot summer months, keep blotting papers close by. My favorite technique: wrap one paper around a non-latex sponge and blot away!

＊ When protecting, cleaning, moisturizing, or exfoliating, don't forget your neck. Your neck needs and deserves loving care, too.

＊ Always try to get eight hours of sleep for healthy, fresh-looking skin.

＊ Put lemon juice on age spots at night to help fade them. Never apply lemon juice to the skin before sun exposure. Citric acid combined with sunshine can cause a burning reaction.

＊ For radiantly beautiful skin, eat foods rich in antioxidants, like blueberries, acacia, and green tea. Also include foods containing omega-3 oils, like salmon and flaxseed.

＊ You cannot shrink pores, but you can keep them clean. Exfoliate gently and well, and then follow with glycolic lotion to keep the sebum at bay.

＊ Clean your makeup brushes every week. Sanitize your makeup bag regularly, too. Your makeup will look

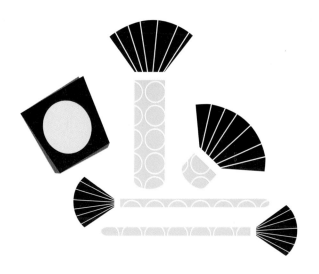

better, and you won't be putting icky, breakout-creating stuff on your skin.

   ✳ Breakouts on the side of your face could indicate it's time to clean the grime from your cell phone. Wipe it down regularly with a little alcohol pad to sweep away bacteria and other zit-creating critters.

   ✳ To moisturize skin during breakouts, apply oil-free moisturizer all over your face and then use a Q-tip to gently wipe it off of the spots. Dip a clean Q-tip into salicylic acid gel and tap it onto the blemishes.

Wacky Rituals

"Elmer's Glue is just as good as a pore strip for removing blackheads from your nose."

—LINDA, 27

"I use Scotch packing tape to remove flaky, dead skin from my face."

—TARYN, 33

"Before bed, I put toothpaste on any zits. They're almost always gone by morning, plus my pillow smells minty-fresh!"

—RACHEL, 25

"An old friend used to eat a papaya every day for breakfast. She would then mix the papaya seeds with cleanser and use the papaya peel as a cloth to wash her face. I haven't tried it, but I do know she had great skin!"

—ERICA, 32

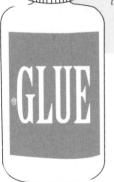

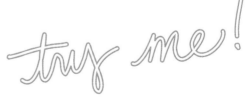

✳ Don't EVER pick at your face. I'm watching you!

✳ Make an appointment with a dermatologist. I swear by mine. Scientifically proven skincare advice from a dermo beats facials, false promises, and foolhardy trends any day. Stop spending on expensive creams and unproven treatments; save up for a yearly dermatological assessment.

✳ Skincare in your teens and twenties is all about prevention. Be diligent about your sunscreen and start moisturizing like mad. If you're oily, choose products that are oil-free or contain salicylic acid to combat breakouts.

✳ Thirtysomething ladies, exfoliation is your skin's best friend. Try microdermabrasion and periodic glycolic peels to keep skin beautiful.

✳ Retinoid creams like Retin-A and Renova are great to start using in your forties: they can help stimulate collagen and diminish fine lines.

✳ To fade age spots or sunspots, see your dermo for a "lunchtime" glycolic peel. It helps lighten up these signs of sun damage and there's no downtime.

✳ Women over fifty can achieve radiant results with dermatologist-prescribed creams. Luminizing face primers are also ideal for you. They bring light to your complexion whether worn under foundation or alone.

✳ Graceful aging always looks lovely, chic, and sophisticated. (Doubt me? Google pictures of the artist Georgia O'Keeffe in her eighties.) If you're going to try fillers, Botox, or plastic surgery, think twice and do half as much. Doing too much detracts from your true beauty and fools no one.

Budget Beauty

TIPS FROM LADIES LIKE YOU!

....

"Cut cleansing pads in half. They're loaded with so much product, much of it goes to waste. By going halfsies, you get twice as many cleansings out of each box!"

—EMILY, 25

"I use food-grade coconut oil as an overnight moisturizer: it has antiviral and antibacterial properties."

—JENNIFER, 37

"Jojoba oil is a great makeup remover and moisturizer booster during the drying winter months. Instead of buying a new bottle, I just add a few drops of jojoba oil to my regular moisturizer. I have acne-prone skin, but this trick does not make me break out."

—ANNA, 25

"To smooth the neck and décolletage area, I like to mix brown sugar with my body wash in the shower."

—HEATHER, 32

"I mix turmeric powder (found in the spice aisle), clay powder, and milk to make a mask. It helps with blemishes and evens out my skin tone. I also take one teaspoon orally with honey to give my skin a glow from the inside out!"

—GUNJAN, 28

"Potato water! Cover your head with a towel and lean your face over a steaming bowl of hot potato water. It makes your skin feel healthy and more vibrant."

—NIRVANA EVELYN, 17

"Here's a great exfoliating technique for very dry skin. Combine sweet almond oil (from a health food store) with crushed almonds (put the cheapest ones you can find in your blender and hit "pulse") to create a paste. Apply to face (excluding eye area) and décolletage, using circular motions. Let the mixture dry on your skin for about ten to fifteen minutes and then rinse with warm water. What a wake-up!"

—KATHLEEN, 55

✳ Don't pile on a bunch of different creams. If you mix a vitamin C cream with alpha hydroxy, for example, you can end up with irritated skin, rashes, and breakouts. Again, a dermo can guide you to the one best product for your unique skin's condition and needs. *Quality*—not quantity—ladies!

 ✳ Sensitive-skinned gals, stay away from anything containing fragrance or anti-aging ingredients like alpha hydroxy, glycolic acids, or retinols. Talk to your dermo to see what is best for you.

 ✳ To test products for sensitivity, apply a bit on your inner elbow. Wait a few hours to see if it's OK for your skin.

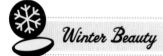

Winter Beauty

During a harsh winter, avoid getting a red, chapped, sore nose by applying a little lip balm around your nostrils before heading outside.

 ✳ Keep an atomizer of water handy to spritz on skin that feels dry or tired.

 ✳ If you want stunning, luminous skin, keep alcohol and caffeine to a minimum. Too much of either will dehydrate your system and leach away B vitamins, resulting in dry, thin skin.

The Nasties

HANGOVERS

As soon as you wake up, start chugging water and keep drinking—ahem, water!—throughout the day. Plain fluids help reduce facial puffiness and counter the dehydrating effects of alcohol.

Pop a wet washcloth into the freezer before you step into a cold shower. Yes, I said cold: you need to stimulate your whole droopy self. After the shower, lie down with the chilled washcloth over your eyes to reduce puffiness.

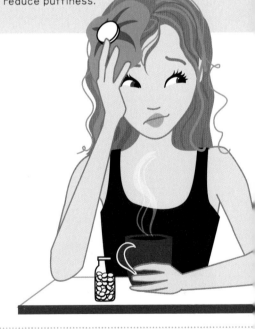

Apply luminizing face primer to instantly restore radiance lost at the party the night before.

To make your eyes look as alert as possible, try adding a little dab of white shimmer powder on the inside tear duct and under the brow bone.

Add a healthy dose of navy blue mascara. A deep navy shade gives eyes a brighter, more awake appearance.

A pop of pink on the apples of the cheeks and on the lips gives the illusion of a fresh face even when you're feeling plowed under.

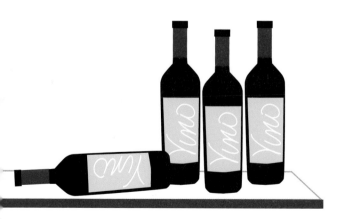

✳ Take your vitamins—especially E, C, A, and other antioxidants that help skin stay gorgeous. Down 'em with plenty of water. H_2O keeps all of your restorative systems running at full power.

✳ Do not smoke if you want smooth, healthy skin. I quit puffing and so can you!

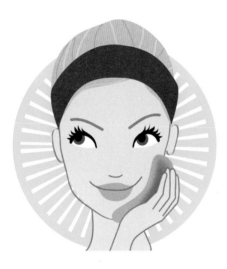

✳ When scheduling a professional facial, be sure to go at least two if not three days before a big event. Give your skin plenty of time to adjust. You don't want to be red-faced on the red carpet!

The Nasties

BIRTHMARKS

To cover a birthmark, use a non—latex sponge to stipple on a yellowish shade of concealer. (Stippling is when you push the sponge into the skin in dabbing motions.) Next, stipple on your flesh—toned concealer. Dust with a translucent powder to set the makeup—providing coverage that lasts all day or night.

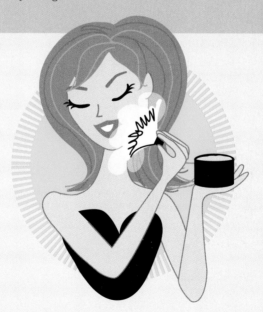

Wacky Rituals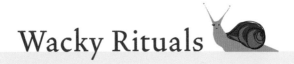

"My grandmother taught me that snail slime helps eliminate acne. Sometimes I secretly wipe a bit on my blemishes. I swear it works!"

—CHERI, 37

"Mix two parts lemon juice to one part Jamaica Rum and pat on freckles."

—DOROTHY RUTLEDGE,
Natural Beauty Secrets (1969)

I suppose you can drink what's left over, and then you won't care whether you have freckles or not!

 Moneysaver

Go bananas for moist, smooth skin. Mash up a really ripe banana and smear it all over your clean face. Relax for about fifteen minutes, and then rinse with warm water. Yummy!

"There are all kinds of masks, ranging from the simplest of clay packs to the meat mask. Fresh beef is cut into very thin slices, according to a pattern you should make at home. Cut pieces of paper—a strip to cover the forehead, another for cheeks, chin, and a thin narrow strip for the nose. Give your pattern to the butcher who will cut the meat accordingly. Leave openings around the eyes and lips. Pack the meat over your skin and secure it with a strip of muslin that has also been cut according to pattern. Leave it on one to two hours or overnight if possible."

—FROM *THE ART OF FEMININE BEAUTY* (1930)

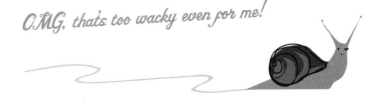

OMG, that's too wacky even for me!

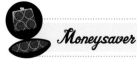

Moneysaver

Use egg white on your face for a quick tightening mask.

Winter Beauty

If a flaky, scaly patch shows up somewhere on your face during the day, dab a bit of lip salve on top to help soothe it away. For overnight care, use a bit of glycolic lotion on the area; it should slough off by morning.

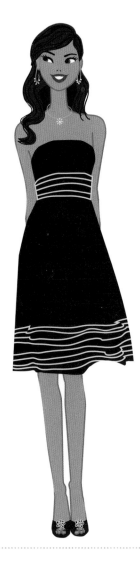

∗ Anti-aging facial exercises are a waste of time. Regular activities give your facial muscles enough of a workout. However, you should be conscious of how you're using your face every day. If you're squinting in the sun instead of wearing sunglasses, that will be detrimental. Commonsense advice: avoid straining your face in any way. Key exception: big smiles. Always a good look!

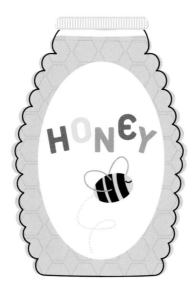

✳ Honey makes a great—if sticky—mask. After applying, lay a hot washcloth over your face to steam the honey into your skin. After ten minutes, wash it off with warm water. Honey's hydrating properties leave your skin feeling super-supple.

✳ Apply a little vitamin K cream on very dark under-eye circles to diminish the bruised look.

Tip Me, Carmindy

Q: *"Do you really need to change up your moisturizer/ cleansing routine each season?"*

—ERIKA, 32

A: *If the weather changes where you live, yes, you do. Summer's humidity calls for an oil-reducing cleanser and lighter moisturizers. Dry winter skin craves richer cleansing and moisturizing formulas, eye cream, and a thick lip balm*

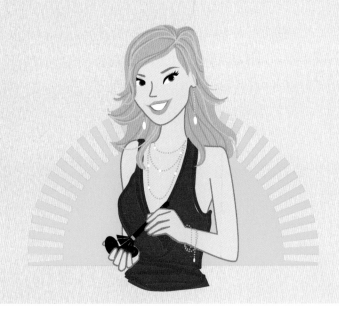

at night. With these switches, your skin will be smooth and fresh in every season.

Q: "After a long illness, my skin became supersensitive. How should I handle my abundant facial hair? Bleaching and waxing are too harsh. I now shave and get razor burn. What to do?"

—DIANE, 49

A: Talk to a dermatologist about permanent hair-removal laser treatments. Better to do it once and never have to go there again.

Q: "Every time I wax my upper lip, I get pink bumps similar to pimples. Threading did this, too. What can I do to combat this problem? Otherwise I have very clear skin. Frustrating!"

—HEATHER, 32

A: You can try bleaching. If your hair is very fine, consider a facial-hair razor. If it's heavier hair, look into permanent hair removal by a trained dermatologist. No fly-by-night "clinics," please.

Q: *"In these tight financial times, how can I try new skincare products? I never know how my skin will react and don't want to throw money out the window."*

—JOYCE, 58

A: Look in magazines for skincare sample packets attached to advertisements. Ask drugstore clerks about available samples. Skincare company websites often give away promotional samples. Beauty blogs also are great resources to see what other women are saying about their experiences with new products.

Q: *"Because of smoking, I have lots of vertical wrinkles. I've tried softening them with fillers, but they're still visible. Any suggestions on how to make them go away?"*

—ELLEN, 61

A: If you haven't yet stopped, stop smoking now! Continue with the fillers; they can take a while to achieve optimum results. Apply a retinoid cream like Renova to help rebuild collagen. Meanwhile, redirect your feature focus: play up your beautiful eyes.

Q: *"Can I use a moisturizer underneath primer?"*

—STEPHANIE, 20

A: *Sure. The moisturizer sinks into your skin, keeping it supple; the primer allows makeup to smooth on evenly.*

Q: *"I'm fair-skinned and have a light beauty mark that sprouts little dark hairs. I'm afraid to use hair-removal products that might cause rashes or burning. What do you recommend?"*

—JOAN, 64

A: *Just pluck it out or have it permanently lasered away by a dermatologist.*

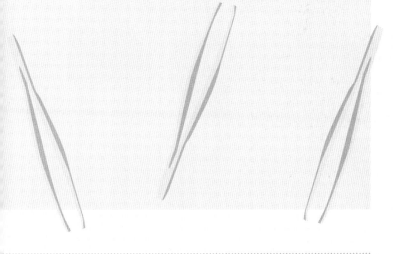

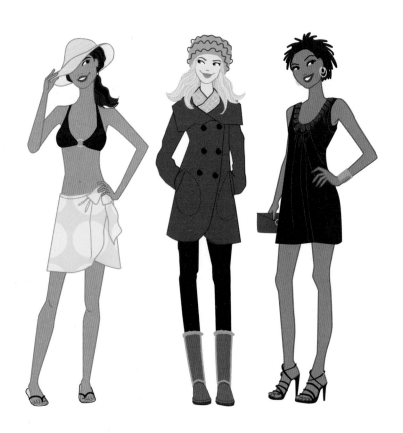

2

Body Basics

Every bit of you can and should radiate beauty. Make a little time each day to care for your whole fine self. Lovely up those elbows and toes. When it comes to pampering, anything—and everything—goes!

To be super-touchable, use a loofah sponge with a good body scrub in the shower. This smoothes the skin and prepares it to drink in your moisturizing lotion.

✳ To lock in moisture, apply body lotion the moment you get out of the shower.

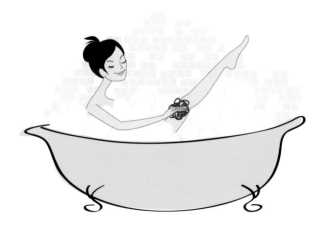

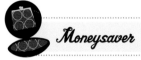

Moneysaver

Create a custom body lotion. Buy a big, inexpensive jug of unscented lotion. Add a few drops of your favorite perfume. Shake it and slather it! For extra gleam, pour a bit of liquid shimmer into your lotion potion.

✳ Sunscreen goes wherever the sun touches your skin—not just your face. Think about your ears, tops of hands, and tops of feet during sandal season. Every exposed inch, every day, ladies!

Summer Beauty

After a dip in the pool, rinse off with clean water or at least spritz your face to remove the chlorine that can dry out your skin. Remember to reapply that sunscreen.

✳ Body-shimmer spray can be used all over for a subtle sheen. Apply it on bare legs to highlight their natural definition. For a sexy, radiant look anytime, try applying a powder version over your chest and arms.

✳ Create stunning shoulders by smoothing shimmering lotion just onto their rounded tops.

✳ Sweep a line of cream shimmer down your bare arms to highlight their shape.

✳ For smooth-looking bare legs, apply a bit of spray foundation. Voilà! No need for stockings.

✳ If your chest skin is red or uneven due to sun damage, apply a little airbrush-style spray foundation and blend in with a non-latex sponge. It goes on lightly and dries quickly; it won't rub off on your clothes. Great for evening looks or anytime you'll be photographed.

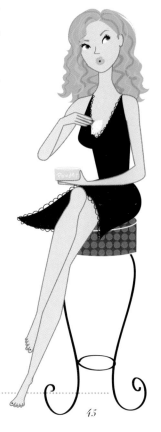

✳ Enhance your cleavage by sweeping a bit of bronzer in between your ta-tas, then apply a highlight shimmer on top of them.

✳ If your chest skin has become a bit crepey, smooth the texture by applying vitamin E, neroli, or argan oil. Seal it in with a moisturizing cream on top.

✳ Rub a little luminizing face primer on your neck and chest for a supersubtle sheen.

Self-tanner 101

Choose a self—tanner that gradually builds color. No carrot—shockers, please! Always exfoliate and shave before application. Afterward, run a cotton swab between your fingers and toes to prevent color from congealing into muddy lines.

If you want a deeper—looking tan, do not apply moisturizer to the skin before a self—tanner. It dilutes the self—tanner and can cause spottiness.

Do apply a spot of moisturizer to ankles, elbows, and knees before using self—tanner. This keeps them from becoming way too dark.

After applying self—tanner, use a moist washcloth to buff knees, elbows, and ankles. Then scrub your hands with a little white sugar. This keeps the tanner from creating dark stains in those crinkly areas.

If you have self—tanner streaks, scrub the dark areas with white sugar in the shower. Then reapply a light new layer of self—tanner into the lighter areas by blending it in with a sponge.

Using self–tanner for an all–over glow can also help you look a few pounds lighter.

Wanna accentuate your muscles? Use self–tanner to contour. After applying a base layer of self–tanner, wait a few hours. Apply a light second layer along the "cut" of your natural muscles.

Be a chest/face matchmaker. If either area is much paler than the other, try building it up to a tonal match by applying a gradual self–tanner.

To extend the lifespan of your self–tan, apply baby oil before stepping out of the shower. This locks in moisture and keeps your skin looking golden longer.

When using self–tanner, avoid body scrubs or facial products like Retin–A, Renova, glycolic acid, or alpha hydroxy. These speed the fade–rate of your tan.

Hot beach babe look! Apply a gold shimmer lotion over a great self–tan.

Banish the muddy bits. If your self–tanner starts looking faded and a little dirty, it's time to scrub with an exfoliant to remove the remaining stain. Let your skin rest at least a day before reapplying.

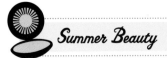

Getting a base tan is ridiculous. You should always fake the bake with self-tanner and use a sunscreen on top to keep your skin protected.

✳ Cream or liquid body bronzer works well if you want a temporary tan that washes off. Be careful not to don light-colored clothing when wearing these body bronzers: they can rub off and stain fabrics.

✳ For subtler warmth, mix body bronzer with a bit of moisturizer before applying.

✳ Tan lines should be considered a mark of shame. A badge of sun damage! Please wear sunscreen, sunshine!

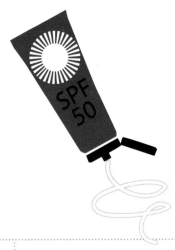

But OK, if you slipped up and now want to slip into a strapless top or dress, here's how to cover the tan lines. Take a non-latex sponge and dip it into a little bronzer. Stipple it into the pale areas for a uniform look.

✳ To conceal blemishes on your chest or shoulders, use a small-tipped concealer brush to dab concealer on the spot. Finish by patting on a little loose powder using a Q-tip.

The Nasties

VARICOSE / SPIDER VEINS

Nothing covers up veins like a little spray foundation sprayed directly onto the legs. These "makeup stockings" erase spiders in a flash.

To exterminate pesky little spider veins, consider laser treatments from a dermatologist. It's easier than you think to just get 'em zapped away for good.

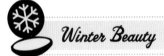

Winter Beauty

Putting a humidifier in your bedroom adds a new dimension to beauty sleep during the cold, dry winter months. Give your parched skin an overnight boost: humidify!

* If your feet get dry and cracked, apply a thick salve or balm, like Vaseline; cover them with warm socks, and head to bed. You'll awaken to dreamily soft tootsies.

* Your elbows, knees, and ankles have almost no oil glands. Keep them hydrated and smooth with extra-rich

moisturizer or balm. Cocoa butter works beautifully as well.

✳ Apply perfume before getting dressed. That way it sinks into your skin, not into your clothes.

✳ If you've laid the perfume on too thick, grab a cotton ball or square and wipe it over your overly spritzed bits to tone down the scent.

✳ Expensive perfume beyond your budget? Try a yummy scented candle. Light it for a bit, blow out the flame, and then drip some wax on your skin. (Be careful, duh! The wax is hot and might burn.) When you rub off the crusty wax, a nice scent is left behind.

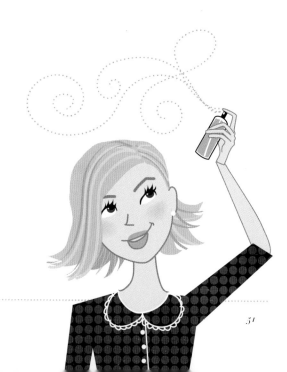

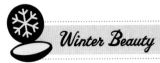

Winter Beauty

Dark-skinned beauties that get ashy during the winter should apply body oils instead of creams for a soft, hydrated look.

* If winter has done a number on your always-cold hands, apply a cream that contains eucalyptus, mint, or rosemary. These botanicals stimulate blood flow—warming your hands while soothing them.

Travel

Forgot your body moisturizer? In a pinch, hair conditioner can eliminate dryness.

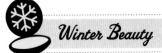

Winter Beauty

Got scaly wintertime elbows? Rub them with sweet almond or coconut oil.

* If your knees, elbows, and heels have become dry and dark, try applying lemon juice to lighten and soften 'em up.

The Nasties

Don't put anything other than disinfectants, healing ointments, and Band—Aids on fresh cuts or scrapes. Kisses are also recommended.

Once a cut or scrape has scabbed over, you can use makeup to hide it. Take a small—tipped concealer brush and trace over the scab with a little mixture of concealer and foundation. Don't follow with powder; it accentuates the scab's dry texture.

To cover fresh, purplish bruises, dab on a little orange—tinted concealer, then add a layer of foundation. If the bruise has faded to yellow, just tap on a skin—matching concealer.

Speed bruises away by applying a healing vitamin K cream to the area.

The Nasties

To hide an unwanted tattoo, first stipple on orange—tinted concealer. Then go over the area again with a skin—matching concealer. The orange layer counters the bluish tones of tattoo ink; the flesh—colored layer can then hide the tattoo.

When stippling concealer onto a tattoo, use a non—latex sponge to dab it over the ink. Always finish with a pat of powder, for long—lasting coverage that won't rub off.

Think fifty times before getting a tattoo, but don't think twice about having one removed with laser treatments from a dermatologist. If you hate your ink, get it zapped. However, don't justify getting a tattoo with the thought that you can laser it off later. Lasers work, but they do not restore skin to its original beauty, nor do they remove every bit of ink. Be cautious!

Crave a new tattoo? Get a henna one at a salon. Henna tattoos last about a week—long enough to satisfy the adornment urge without risking a permanent mistake.

❊ Busty ladies sometimes have trouble with sweat collecting under or between their breasts. Try applying a little deodorant or mattifying gel in this area to reduce dampness.

❊ If you are on antihistamines or use Retin-A–type prescriptions, be careful when waxing. Your skin is likely to now be more delicate and rip-prone. To avoid injuries and scabs, go easy.

❊ Listen up! Your ears need attention. Don't forget to lavish moisturizer on your lovely lobes.

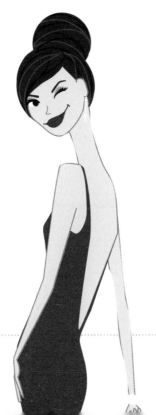

Budget Beauty

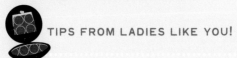

TIPS FROM LADIES LIKE YOU!

"Fabulous cornmeal scrub recipe. Mix one cup cornmeal, one cup honey, one and one-half cups heavy whipping cream. Refrigerate overnight so the cream gets absorbed. About an hour before use, take it out and let it stand at room temperature. After a long soak or hot shower, scrub it all over your body—avoiding the face. Rinse, moisturize, and voilà! Amazingly soft skin that smells delicious!"

—SARAH, 36

"I have a small bathroom with a pedestal sink. To create counter space during my beauty routine, I put a polypropylene cutting board over the sink bowl. Spills can be easily washed away and it stores nicely when I'm finished."

—STACIA, 24

"Before bedtime, smear your hands with Vaseline. Then place them in plastic bags followed by big socks. Sleep in these 'mittens' for a deep moisturizing treatment."

—DIANE, 55

"I apply baby oil on my décolletage, shoulders, and arms to create a sleek, sexy, and more toned look in evening wear."

—LISA, 37

"The night before a pageant (or big event), we'd rub Preparation H cream (not the gel) on our stomachs and thighs and then wrap 'em in Saran Wrap. The next morning they'd look tighter."

—TONI, 38

"I put a light, inexpensive olive oil in a small plastic bottle that won't break in the shower. I add a few drops of my favorite essential oil to give it a yummy scent. At the very end of my shower, I smooth this mixture all over my body, neck, and face. Rinse a bit, and then pat myself dry. I follow with lotion to stay supersoft."

—VICTORIA, 57

"After polishing my nails, I open the freezer door and stick my nails by the vents where the cold air blows to dry them quickly. It really prevents smudges, especially in the humid summer months."

—PATRICIA, 59

"Cosmetology schools offer great beauty services at great rates. I prefer getting my manicures and pedicures done at schools because students are very good about sanitizing their equipment."

—JENNY, 53

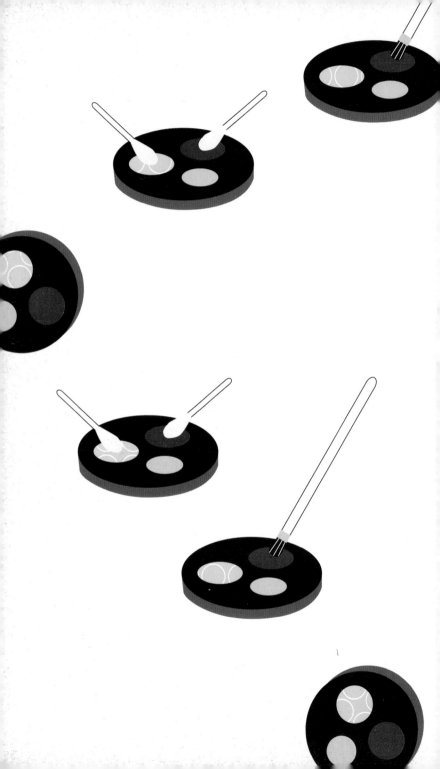

3

Laying the Foundation:

Skin Makeup

You've heard me say it a thousand times: makeup should enhance your natural beauty, not mask it. That goes *double* for foundation, concealer, powder, and all the other tools we use to create radiant-looking skin.

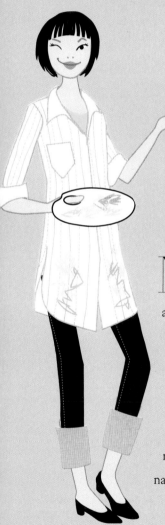

Never be a slave to your prettifying products. With a light touch and a positive attitude, makeup can and should be your happy little servant! Use these tips to serve up a smooth, glowing complexion.

For the lightest coverage, smooth on a tinted moisturizer. This protects, moisturizes, and covers in one go for a natural-looking glow.

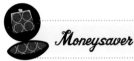

Moneysaver

Create your own tinted moisturizer by simply mixing foundation with an SPF-infused moisturizer and blending it in.

  ∗ Apply a luminizing face primer before foundation to even out your skin's texture and create a perfectly smooth canvas for your makeup.

  ∗ When shopping for your perfect foundation, choose three shades that closely match your skin. Apply all three next to each other along your jawline. The one that best blends into your skin is your perfect pick.

  ∗ Never use the inside of the wrist to test foundation shades. Always use the jawline area and take the chest into consideration. Sometimes your face and chest are different shades. Adjust your choices so the total effect looks polished. Avoid the dreaded demarcation lines!

✳ When choosing foundation shades, always steer clear of really pinky undertones. The slightest yellow undertone is more universally flattering.

✳ Some darker-skinned women have varying skin tones around their faces. I like to choose the shade that falls in between these two shades and blend for a unifying effect. Or pick two shades of foundation and blend them on the appropriate areas for a balanced look.

✳ When you're changing up your wardrobe, think about adjusting your makeup, too. You should buy a fall/winter shade of foundation to match your face and body when you are at your palest and a spring/summer shade to match you when you are bronzed from self-tanners.

✳ Oily-skinned gals should use spray or oil-free liquid foundations. Cream or powder foundations are too heavy and masking for you.

✳ To reduce oiliness, try applying mattifying gels or serums before your foundation to control shine throughout the day.

✳ Dry and normal-skinned ladies fare best with liquid foundations or tinted moisturizers.

✳ Most mature women fare best with liquid foundations. Skip thick pancake or powder foundations: they settle into fine lines.

✳ If you want to skip foundation but still have a healthy-looking glow, try a facial self-tanner to warm up your complexion.

✳ Whenever possible, apply foundation in natural daylight to ensure a perfectly seamless finish.

✳ Foundation Application Fundamentals: Fingers lay it on a bit heavier; so does a foundation brush. Using a non-latex sponge creates lighter coverage.

✳ For sheer-looking coverage, blend foundation on in sweeping and blending motions. For areas needing more coverage, stipple it on by pushing the foundation into the skin using a blotting motion.

✳ Always apply spray foundation with a non-latex sponge. Never spray it directly on the face: it looks too heavy and can cover brows and lashes.

✳ For a sheer, natural finish, put a bit of primer or moisturizer on your non-latex sponge along with the foundation. This combo lightens up the coverage.

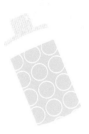

* Many women don't need a full face of foundation. Unevenness tends to happen around the central part of the face, like around the eyes, nose, and chin. Focus your foundation here and blend out toward the cheeks.

* If you prefer a full foundation application, make sure you blend into the hairline and down the neck a bit to avoid demarcation lines. Try using a clean sponge to buff makeup into these areas for a flawless finish.

* If you hate the feel of foundation, just spot-conceal where necessary for a no-makeup look.

* After applying foundation, use a clean non-latex sponge to blend over any areas where you tend to get creases: for line-free loveliness that lasts.

* Slathered it on too thick? Use a clean non-latex sponge to blend down excess foundation and buff it to a perfect finish.

✳ If your skin looks too dry after foundation, try spritzing it with a little water. Then blend lightly with a non-latex sponge.

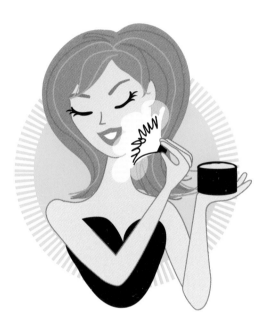

✳ If your foundation looks too light, simply sweep a shimmer-free bronzer all over the skin to deepen the color.

✳ If your foundation looks too dark, try sweeping on a lighter face powder to tone it down. Don't make a habit of the powder trick; go shopping for a better shade, girlfriend.

✴ For a dewy-looking complexion, after you apply your foundation, dab on a bit of highlighter down the bridge of your nose, on top of the cheekbones, and across the forehead.

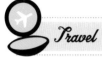

Travel

Quickie make-do foundation: mix a little moisturizer on the back of your hand with a smear of concealer and apply it over the skin with a non-latex sponge.

✴ Fix any afternoon splotches: mix a little moisturizer and foundation, put just a touch on a non-latex sponge, and lightly buff the area until it looks even.

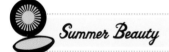

Summer Beauty

Don't wear a full face of foundation at the beach: it's way too heavy. Instead, go for a tinted moisturizer that provides hydration, sun protection, and sheer coverage.

To minimize the look of your pores, first apply a mattifying gel. Next, apply a spray foundation using a non-latex sponge; stipple it on by pushing it into the skin. Then lightly dust on a face powder.

✳ Add a drop of liquid shimmer to your foundation to freshen your complexion. Really nice for a night out!

✳ To warm up a pale face, add a drop of liquid bronzer to your foundation before applying it.

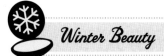

Winter Beauty

Got wintertime drabs? Switch to luminous primers and foundations to combat dull-looking skin.

✳ Toss any foundation you've had sitting around for over a year. Formulas can degrade after air enters the packaging. Besides, if you haven't used it up in a year, it's probably not working for you!

✳ Don't apply concealer before foundation: you'll just wipe it off as you apply foundation. Always conceal afterward.

✳ Have two types of concealers at the ready: a lighter shade for under-eye darkness and a foundation-matching shade to cover spots, veins, or blemishes.

✳ If you're fair-skinned, correct under-eye darkness by blending on sheer light pink concealer: it helps bounce light off the dark areas, brightening the face.

✳ If you have medium skin tone, reduce under-eye darkness by dabbing on a peachy beige concealer to brighten up the area.

✳ A golden beige concealer helps eliminate under-eye darkness for darker skin tones.

✳ To attack extremely dark circles, pat on a mixture of your under-eye concealer and your blemish concealer. Blend it well and with a gentle touch.

✳ I like to use my ring finger to dab on brightening concealer under the eyes. It is the weakest digit, so won't pull too hard on that delicate eye area.

✳ When choosing concealer for blemishes, don't use a shade much lighter than your foundation. It will highlight rather than conceal. Instead, pick a foundation-matching concealer with a slightly thicker consistency for staying power.

✳ When hiding an age spot or a blemish, always use a small-tipped concealer brush to place a little concealer on the area. Use the brush to then lightly blend the edges so it disappears into the skin. Set with a touch of powder.

✳ If you don't have concealer handy, cover spots or blemishes with a little foundation using a small-tipped concealer brush. Use foundation left over in the cap or on the nozzle. It's a little thicker and can be lightly layered onto spots.

✳ To conceal a really dark spot or pit on the skin, try dabbing it with a blemish concealer one shade lighter than your foundation to even things out.

✳ If your spot concealer is too thin, try mixing in a touch of face powder. This thickens it so you can achieve fuller coverage.

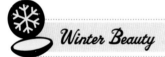

Winter Beauty

If concealer or foundation around your eyes becomes thick and cakey late in the day, simply tap a little eye cream on top of the area with your finger to soften it a bit. Then blend it down with a non-latex sponge or Q-tip.

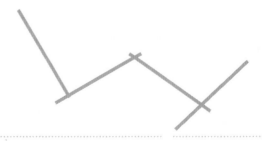

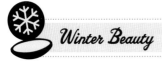

Winter Beauty

Does Jack Frost turn your skin red? Apply a calming skin cream; follow with your foundation. Next, pat yellow-tinted concealer over the reddest areas to tone them down.

✳ Feed your skin as you enhance it. Choose products packed with antioxidant ingredients and vitamins for a healthy-looking complexion.

✳ Don't use dark contour powders or creams to heavily shade the face; it always looks unnatural. If you absolutely must shade an area that just drives you crazy, sweep on a bit of shimmer-free bronzer.

The Nasties

To help fade melasma, apply a cream containing hydroquinone or kojic acid. Used consistently, these ingredients fade dark spots over time. Be sure to stay out of the sun and wear a high-SPF sunscreen. Sun savvy will also help keep the melasma from reappearing.

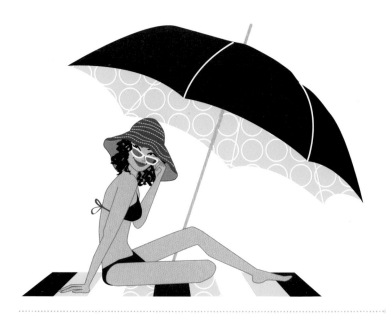

* Use highlighter to show off your face's beautiful planes. If you use cream highlighter, apply it after your foundation. If you use powder highlighter, apply it after face powder.

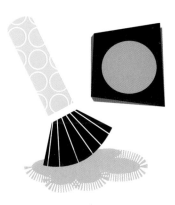

* Dab a brightening concealer cream (like one used under the eyes) along the nasal labial folds around the mouth to minimize "smile line" creases.

* Face powder should go on after foundation, concealer, and cream blush, but before other powder products, like powder blush or bronzer.

* The main purpose of powder is to set makeup and eliminate shine. A little shine keeps skin looking fresh, so choose translucent powders and apply mostly to the T-zone.

✳ Finely milled translucent face powder zaps shine without depositing a lot of powder on the skin. Stay away from heavily pigmented colored powders that add a heavy extra layer and make skin look dull.

✳ Apply a yellow-tinted sheer face powder over foundation to tone down redness in ruddy skin.

✳ For oil slicks during the day, use blotting papers to zap unwanted shine. If you just keep powdering, you end up looking cakey.

✳ For a naturally dewy look, skip face powder altogether. I'm not a fan of using more than the minimum powder necessary, no matter what look you're after!

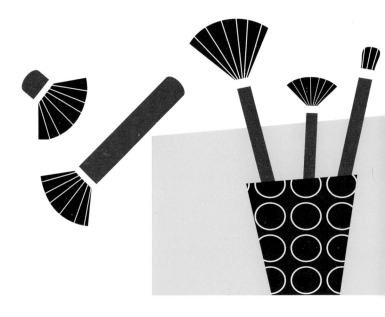

✳ Pressed powders are best for touchups on the go; for your morning makeup, choose loose powders.

✳ Apply loose powder using a blush brush, not a big poofy powder brush. Always tap off excess powder before applying it to the skin. This ensures light coverage—avoiding an avalanche!

✳ With pressed powder, never wipe the puff across the powder and then smear all over your skin. You'll smudge your foundation. Instead, lightly dab the puff into the pressed powder and then blot the skin lightly with it. Be sure you wash-n-dry your puffs regularly, too.

✳ If you have applied too much powder, take a big clean fluffy powder brush and sweep away the excess.

✳ Avoid using much powder around the crows'-feet area of the eyes: it can accentuate wrinkles.

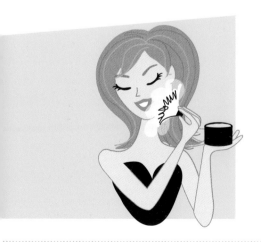

The Nasties

ROSACEA

Women with rosacea, you can tame the flame with makeup and a few new habits. With makeup, first apply foundation to your whole face. Next, stipple a bit more foundation onto your red areas—pushing it into the skin, not sweeping it across. Finish with a yellow—tinted light powder to counteract any remaining redness.

To neutralize stubbornly red areas, tap on yellow—tinted concealer after your foundation. Finish with yellow—tinted powder.

With your natural rosy flush, you can skip blush. Spend your blush money instead on a fabulous new lip color!

Facial scrubs can irritate rosacea—affected skin. To exfoliate dryness, lightly rub a tiny bit of facial scrub on unaffected areas. Do not attempt to exfoliate any red patches.

Stay away from steam baths or facials. Heat treatments exacerbate the redness caused by rosacea.

Steer clear of red wine and spicy foods: they can cause capillaries to swell and redden. Please do, however, keep that spicy personality of yours running hot!

Glamazon

Evening glowing-goddess look: after foundation, concealer, and powder, dust a very sheer application of loose pale gold shimmer across the face.

* Bronzer is a great way to sweep on that just-back-from-vacation freshness. But don't get crazy. Bronzer should never be more than a few shades darker than your usual skin tone.

* The best bronzers for oily or combo-skinned gals are gels, powders, and sprays. Ladies with drier skin should try bronzer creams and sticks.

* Apply bronzer starting at the temples. Blend it down the sides of the face by the hairline and then sweep a bit under the cheeks. Go lightly when brushing across the forehead, nose, and chin or you'll look more grubby than gorgeous.

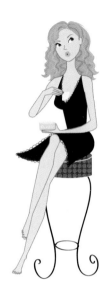

＊ If you're bronzing, try a hint on the neck and chest as well as the face for an even, polished look.

＊ To minimize jowls, apply a bit of shimmer-free cream or powder bronzer to the area.

＊ Shimmery bronzer can highlight fine lines. Older skin achieves a better glow from self-tanners or shimmer-free bronzers.

＊ When using bronzer or self-tanner, use little or no face powder; tanned skin looks muddy with powder piled on top.

＊ Never cover up your freckles. They are beautiful!

Summer Beauty

Fight the sweaty summer sloppies. Control shine and keep oil at bay by applying a mattifying gel; follow with oil-free foundation. Dab a little mattifying gel on your eyelids as well; it keeps eye shadow from slipping off. Finish with a light dusting of translucent powder. Keep blotting papers nearby for touch-ups. Your complexion will be glowing, not greasy.

Tip Me, Carmindy

Q: "I am a fair-skinned, freckle-faced brunette who wears foundation and concealer. However, my neck and décolletage are naturally ruddy and blotchy, so they appear to be an entirely different skin tone, especially in lower-cut evening clothes. Add a glass of wine and forget about it! What's a girl to do?"

—ANNE, 52

A: Spray a light mist of airbrush spray foundation on the neck and chest area and blend lightly with a sponge. Once dry, spray foundations won't rub off on clothes. For a more permanent solution, ask a dermatologist about peels or laser treatments that can even out blotchiness.

Q: "I have a red nose. Despite cream foundation and concealer, my nose still pinks its way through! It's gotten especially bad now that I'm pregnant. If I put on even a light dusting of blush, it looks like a pink swath across the center of my face. What to do?"

—ERYNNE, 26

A: Dab on a little yellow-tinted concealer right after your foundation application. Dust on a little yellow-tinted powder to set it. This yellowish shade helps neutralize any redness.

Q: "I used to have a bad habit of picking at my acne. I stopped, but still have very dark scars all around my face. Is there a way to cover them up all day without using over-greasy concealer?"

—JASMYN, 18

A: Try a fade cream at night. During the day dab a sheer, oil-free concealer into the scars using a small-tipped concealer brush for precise placement.

Q: "What's the trick to using mineral foundation? It just does not seem to work as well as liquid for me and I am sure it is because I do not apply it properly."

—ELLEN, 61

A: I'm not a fan of mineral makeup for most women. I think liquid foundation works better on most gals, because the color and coverage remain intact all day. If you do use mineral makeup, be sure not to apply it too heavily, as it can be a bit chalky. Take the time to blend it well with a brush, twirling in circular motions.

Q: "How do you cover up forehead lines without making them stand out that much more? I use foundation, but they are still very visible."

—DENISE, 48

A: First, apply a luminizing face primer to bounce light off this area. Then smooth a very sheer layer of foundation. Blend it down well, especially around the lines so that any excess does not accumulate there.

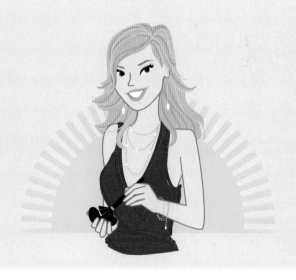

Date Makeup

Guys usually don't like to see (or kiss!) a lot of makeup on their favorite lady. If you want to make a **GRAND STATEMENT**, go for a **bold** eye look. Just don't scare the poor boy!

Up your kiss—me odds: keep lipstick and gloss neutral and light. Dark or goopy lips don't tempt many suitors.

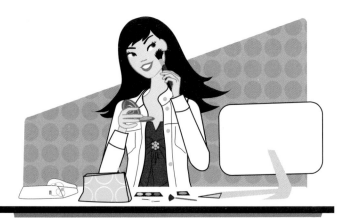

Try a *flavored* lip formula every once in a while to surprise your love bug. Sweetness shared is sweetness doubled!

You can't go wrong with my Five-minute Face. Lightly apply foundation, concealer, and powder. Use a little highlight under the eyebrow (on the brow bone under the arch) and on the inside corners of the eye. Apply a little eyeliner along the upper lash line and mascara on the upper lashes. Add a pop of blush and a light-tinted lip balm.

You're ready to roll.

The Nasties

PASSION RASH

Making out with beard—bristly boys can be fun; it can also scrape off a fine layer of skin from your chin and cheeks . . . ouch! Help your crush rash heal by applying a little cortisone cream; it soothes away the redness. Use your fingers to lightly dab a little liquid foundation on top to conceal any remaining evidence!

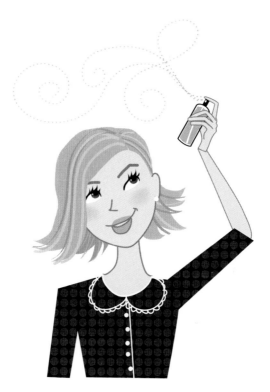

✳ With perfume, spray above your head and let the fragrance "fall" into your hair. This way he'll get a subtle sniff of scent, not an overbearing wallop.

✳ Impromptu after-work date? Take your look from day to night in a flash. Blot away excess oil with blotting papers. Conceal any redness and buff away any foundation smears. Add dark eyeliner and a deeper evening shade of eye shadow. Sweep on a bit more highlighter and a light application of translucent powder. Slick on sexy lip gloss. Now go charm your cubicle mate!

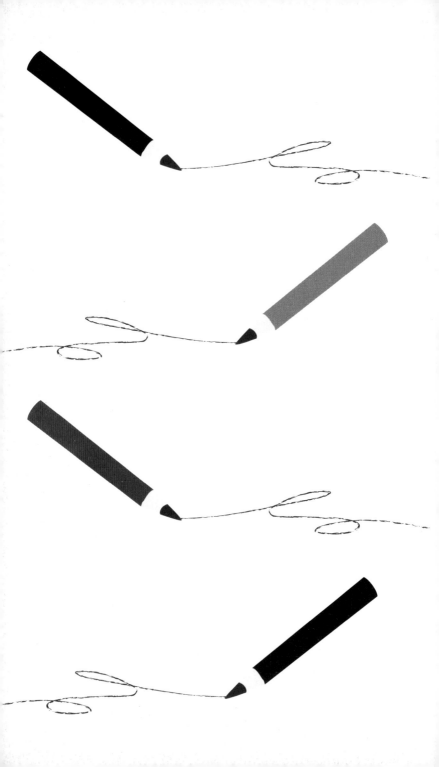

4

Brows
That Wow

Oh, these glorious arches frame the face and bring definition to the windows of your soul. Sleek, elegant eyebrows are within your reach. Here's how to get your brows in tip-top shape!

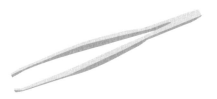

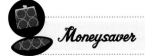 *Moneysaver*

Tame brows with a clean toothbrush; it's cheaper than a brow comb but works just as well.

 * Applying a light slick of Vaseline over the brows will give them a healthy-looking shine.

 * Brows should be naturally flowing, uniform arches and not little squares with tails. The paisley look is so not pretty.

 * In general, thicker brows work for ladies with prominent bone structure; thinner brows enhance smaller-framed faces.

 * Over-tweezed brows age a face. Mature ladies should keep a nice healthy shape, skip the anorexic plucking, and fill brows in a bit if need be.

✳ To avoid disasters, go for a professional shaping every three to four weeks. All you have to do is pluck the strays that pop up between visits.

✳ If you have fine brows, tweezing is the way to go. Plucking allows you to take out one or two hairs at a time, giving you more control.

✳ If your brows are a bit heavier, waxing is a good choice. Waxing allows more hairs to be removed at once—meaning less time and less pain for you. When choosing an aesthetician, make sure you see her waxing handiwork on someone else first to ensure you like her style.

✳ If you have very hairy brows or if they grow down from the hairline, threading—an ancient technique from India—could be ideal for you. I'm always amazed at how flawless a woman's brow looks after threading. Those twirling threads remove many hairs very quickly; the results are perfect.

✳ If your brows grow straight down, use a curved pair of cuticle scissors and snip them from underneath into perfect shape.

✳ Always start your grooming routine by brushing the brow hairs straight up with a spooly brush, which looks just like a clean mascara wand. Trim any long, wild hairs with a pair of cuticle scissors.

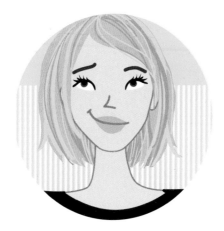

✳ Stay away from brow stencils. Everyone's brow bone is unique. Stenciling on a "standardized" brow will look ridiculous. It's like wearing someone else's hairpiece.

✳ If you want to pluck a perfect brow but have no idea where to begin, take a white eyeliner pencil and draw the ideal shape over your existing brows then pluck around the drawn-on stencil. Step back and see if that's the brow look you're after.

✳ You need two sets of tweezers. A slant tip for pulling many thicker hairs at once and a pair of fine, needle-nose-tipped tweezers for getting the little, hard-to-reach ones.

✳ The best place to pluck your brows is in front of a sunny window. Wave at the neighbors!

✳ If your eyesight is poor, use a 10x magnification mirror to really see the little buggers.

Shaping 101:

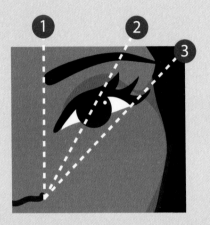

FIND YOUR BROW'S STARTING POINT. Rest a brow brush along the side of your nose horizontally. Where the top of the brush passes across your forehead is where your brow should begin. Map out the other side as well and pluck all the hairs in between these two "unibrow" points.

MAP OUT YOUR ARCH. If you hold a brow brush along the side of your nose and angle it across your iris, where it passes across the brow is where it should arch. Pluck the strays under this area for a natural—looking arch. Please pluck only a few at a time; step away to evaluate so you don't go overboard.

* Don't pluck too often, because the roots of your brows may become stunted and they will never grow back. You really need to take your time and consider what hairs you could permanently live without.

* Clean up stray hairs above the brow to keep them looking sleek and clean. It's an old myth that you should not pluck above the brow. If you're fuzzy, go for it!

* If you want your eyes to appear wider, pluck a few hairs closer toward the inner corners by the sides of the bridge of your nose.

* If you want your eyes to appear closer together, allow the hairs toward the bridge of the nose to grow closer together.

* If you are older, shorten your brow a bit at the ends. Long, extended brows can cause a droopy eye effect.

＊ Beware of the little fuzzies. Pluck the fine, almost invisible, little hairs that sometimes grow on the lid under the brow, especially on fair-haired gals. If you don't, highlight shadow will catch on them and look rather chalky. Remove the fine hairs and the highlight will look clean and perfect.

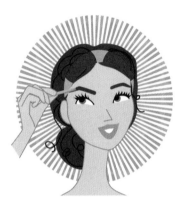

＊ To minimize pain, pluck right after a hot shower. The follicles will be more open and hairs will come out easier.

＊ To ease your tweezing, pull the skin taut, grab the hairs at the base as close to the skin as you can get, and gently pull.

＊ Always pull hairs in the direction that they grow. If you pull them in the wrong direction they may start to grow out that way or become ingrown.

＊ If your brows grow straight out, take a hand mirror and go stand in front of a sunny window. Turn your head sideways. Out of the corner of your eye look for and snip any hairs that stick out more than a quarter of an inch. Then fill in the brow with a bit of brow color. To keep brows lying down, apply a bit of brow wax.

✳ Anbesol or any topical pain cream can be applied before tweezing to make the going easier.

✳ If your skin becomes irritated and red after a plucking, try a cold compress and some soothing aloe gel.

✳ Use a brightening concealer around the eyes after plucking. It reduces any redness while highlighting your new perfect shape.

✳ If you have over-plucked your brows, confront the situation like a bad haircut. You gotta grow 'em out. Leave them be for about three months and then start from scratch. I know, the growing-out process will make you crazy (like a bad bangs job), but just hang in there!

✳ A pencil is the easiest tool for filling in your brows. Make sure it is sharp; then lightly feather it on for a natural look. If the pencil is dull or if you push too hard, brows will have that artificial, drawn-on look.

✳ When using a liquid brow color, apply in small, featherlike strokes with a stiff angle brush to fill in sparse eyebrows.

Brilliant Brows!

Most Asian brows need a little filling in, as they tend to be on the sparse side. I prefer using a stiff angled brush to feather the brow color downward from the tops of the brow for a clean look.

Blondes should choose a brow shade the same color as the darkest strand of their hair. It adds definition to their eyes.

If you have gray hair, use a taupe brow color. It frames your eyes better than a gray shade. Gray looks too dull on the skin.

If you are a true redhead, sable is your perfect fill—in shade. Straight red looks a little strange.

Brunettes should choose a brow color one shade lighter than their hair color. It looks softer on their skin.

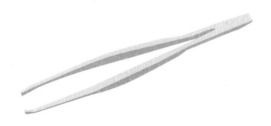

✳ For a very chic look, extend your brows about a quarter-inch at the ends, using pencil or brow corrector. This gives your eyes an elongated elegance.

✳ As we age, brows can become sparse and fade a bit. Fill in mature brows with a little brow color to ensure your eyes always stand out.

✳ If you have a gap in your brows due to a scar, buy, at an art-supply store, a tiny little brush with a few long hairs in it. Use this to paint on a few strokes of liquid brow corrector. This creates a flawless, hairlike result.

✳ If you have filled in your brows too much, take a small-tipped concealer brush dipped into a little foundation and feather it through the brows very lightly to soften the color.

✳ After you apply your foundation, always take a clean Q-tip and sweep it over your eyebrows to remove any foundation residue for a nice, clean arch.

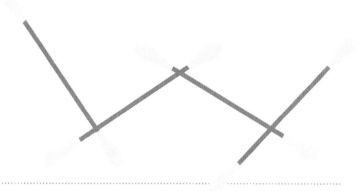

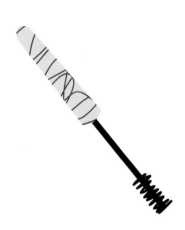

✳ Brow powder is best used for a natural-looking brow but can get a little chalky. Follow it with a clear brow gel.

✳ For brow color that stays in place through heat, humidity, and even swimming, go for a waterproof brow corrector.

✳ For brows that just won't stay put, apply a brow gel after you fill brows in to keep them in place.

✳ Before you apply brow gel, wipe off any excess with a paper towel. If you apply too much, it can dry up and flake like dandruff. Yuck!

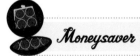

Moneysaver

Regular hair gel applied with a little spooly brush can work just like brow gel.

* For a sexy outdoorsy look, brush the thickest part of your brows (near the inside corner) straight up and apply a clear brow gel.

* A tinted brow gel is the lightest and most natural way to keep brows in place and add a hint of color at the same time.

* Brow wax is the best product to use for stubborn brows that won't stay in place.

Glamazon

For a superchic evening look, pair a red lip with a brow that has been filled in perfectly with a tad more brow color than usual.

* If you're blond, apply a bit of gold shimmer powder over brows for a beautiful evening highlight.

* If you have dramatically changed your hair color, change your brow color product or ask your colorist to touch up your brows to match.

* Do not pull out gray or white brow hairs. It can cause gaps you'll have to spend extra time filling in. Opt instead for a professional dye job.

Budget Beauty

TIPS FROM LADIES LIKE YOU!

"I discovered dyeing my own eyebrows. At first I used hair dye kits for women. But those ran $10 a box, and I wasted most of the product. Then I discovered men's dye kits (for beards). You can squeeze out just what you need. Am happy to say I have been on the same box of dye for the last eighteen months."

—SHERRI, 43

"In a pinch, use a No. 2 pencil to fill in blond eyebrows."

—JAIME, 22

"Before I do anything with my brows (whether shaping/tweezing or applying brow-defining products), I raise my eyebrows as high as I can. I put my index fingers on the high-est part of my arch, then I will push down as hard as I can with my forehead muscles against my fingers. I hold this for about ten seconds. It always seems to make my arch more defined for a minute or so in order for me to do my thing. The result: a perfectly groomed eyebrow every time!"

—JENNIFER, 30

"Use a slick of ChapStick over the brows to keep them in place if you don't have brow gel."

—GINA, 27

✳ To conceal one or two white brow hairs, paint a bit of waterproof liquid brow corrector or liquid liner over the top.

✳ If you have given yourself a botched brow job, fill them in the best you can until they grow out. Then draw attention to your mouth with a fabulous new lip color!

✳ Lighter brows look better on older skin. Lighten up a shade every decade after forty.

✳ Jolene's Cream Bleach is a great simple product for lightening brows. Though it's mainly used for unwanted facial hair, Jolene's can also lighten up brows a shade or two in a flash.

✳ If you have bumps after a brow wax, stay away from shimmer highlighter under the brow. It can accentuate the rough spots.

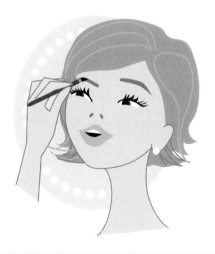

✳ DO NOT permanently tattoo your brows—or anything else on your face! It never looks natural. The ink eventually fades to a purplish color and your brows may droop over time. Your permanent arch may wind up in another location. Not a good look!

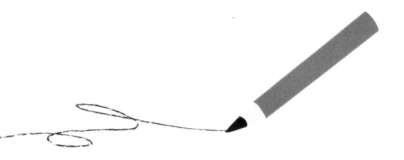

Tip Me, Carmindy

Q: *"A few years ago, my eyebrows began growing straight out from the arch to the outside point. Yikes! I don't know whether I should pluck them out or trim them back. I'll still have hairs growing straight out, but they'll be shorter if I trim them. How to handle these 'senior' brows?"*

—PATSY, 61

A: *Trim them to lie closer to the skin. If they look a bit sparse, simply fill them in with a little brow corrector.*

Q: *"What to do with the pesky white eyebrow hair? My hairdresser refuses to color them. There are simply too many to pluck out without leaving eyebrows sparse."*

—MICHELLE, 45

A: *Ask another colorist to lightly dye your brows to match your hair. Any salon worth a hill of beans can and will do this for you.*

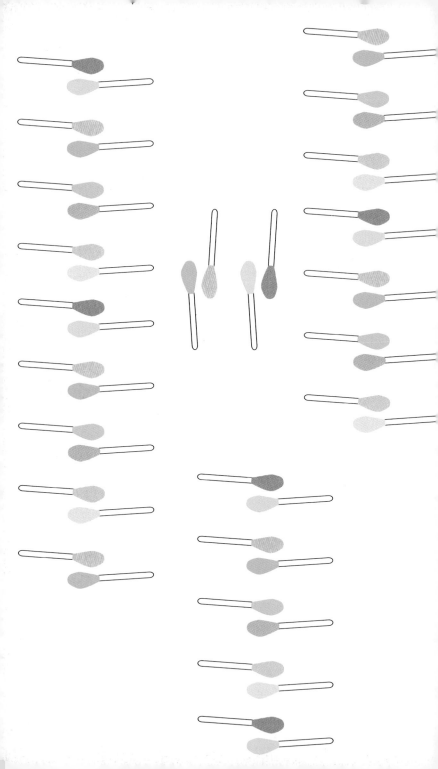

5

Eye
Essentials

Read any good novel and you'll notice how authors describe eyes to inform what's going on with a character: *Her eyes widened, narrowed, blazed, pierced, laughed, shifted, warmed, danced.* Eyes express our emotions—giving others a glimpse at what's stirring under the surface. And what a bountiful bevy that can be! Fascinating creature, do I have some fabulous eye tips for you!

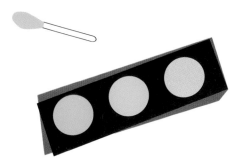

If you want your eyes to really pop, don't match your eye shadow to your eye color. Create greater impact by choosing opposite colors. For example, green eyes—go plum; blues—try brown; browns—head for blues, greens, or plums; hazel—go jade or forest-green. Play with contrast; skip matchy-matchy for the most shazam, madam!

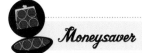

Moneysaver

Foolproof Shadow Shopping: Buy the already coordinated trio compacts. In one purchase, you get a highlight, lid, and contour shade; this darkest shade can also double as eyeliner.

✳ If in doubt, a slightly shimmering brown eye shadow works for every age and skin tone.

✳ Help colors stick and stay true for hours by creating an eye shadow base. Apply a thin veil of foundation and translucent powder on the lids and under the eyes.

✳ Sweep on powder eye shadows instead of creams for more staying power.

✳ Keep a sponge that's been dipped in a little foundation handy. If any shadow falls on the skin during your application, sweep it cleanly away with this "magic eraser."

✳ The most basic way to apply eye shadow is the three-color look. You never need more than three shades on your eyes. Apply a highlight color under the brow and on the inner corners of the eyes; sweep a medium shade across the lid from lash line to crease. Finish with a contour shade swept across the crease.

✳ For a simple-but-defined eye, choose a mid-tone shade and sweep it only from the lash line to the crease. This creates enough depth to skip the eyeliner.

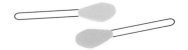

For a fast morning lift, apply highlight shadow under the brow and on the inner corners only. The contrast of the highlight next to your bare skin on the lid creates the illusion you are already wearing a neutral lid shadow.

※ Try just a dab of highlight shadow on the center of the lid to bring some light to your eyes.

※ For a quick eye-brightening look, lightly apply a single highlight shade across the whole eye from lash line to the brow bone. If you have light skin, go for a white, iridescent, or pale pink shade; medium skin try champagne or pale gold; dark skin head for a sunset pinky-gold or pale bronze.

※ Remember that light highlight shades enhance areas and make them stand out, and darker contour shades make areas recede and become more defined.

Wacky Rituals

"When my eyelids get very dry, red, and sting-y, I put Chap-Stick on them before I go to sleep. My eyelids feel great by morning."

—ANNA, 25

"Preparation H gel reduces puffy eyes fast. I let it dry and follow with my moisturizer. It's inexpensive and a tube lasts for ages and ages."

—FRAN, 63

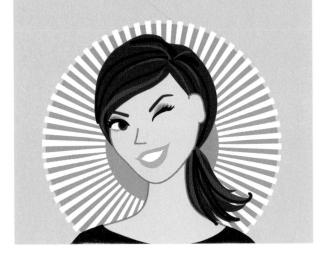

✳ To enhance close-set eyes, apply light highlight shadows on the inner half of the lids.

✳ For far-set eyes, apply darker lid shades on the inner half of the lids.

✳ Ladies with deep-set eyes should avoid using dark contour shades on the lids; those just make them further recede. Instead, play with highlight shades on the lid and mid-tone shades in the crease.

✳ Enhance Asian or hooded eyes by applying mid-tone or contour shades across the entire lid area and up to the crease right under the brow bone.

✳ Big eyes look amazing with contour shades applied across the entire lid from lash line to crease.

✳ Small eyes look great with light, shimmering highlight shades across the lids. Add a little contour shade across the outer half of the crease and along the outer half of the bottom lash line.

✳ To bring out the little gold or copper flecks that occur in some irises, sweep that same shade of shadow along the lid.

✳ Older women do best with sheer, finely milled shadows that have a touch of luminosity. Cream eye shadows can cause buildup in the creases; chalky matte shadows can look parched.

Smokin'
Hot Smoky Eye

To achieve the perfect smoky eye look, you must create a gradation of color. Start by applying the darkest shadow shade on the lid. Place a medium shade in the crease and under the lower lash line. Finish with a pop of highlight shadow under the brow and on the inner corners of the eyes.

Make your smoky eye more chic and sophisticated. Mix shades of gray and black with purple, green, silver, plum, or blue.

Avoid "ash—fall" during your smoky application. Fold a tissue and place it under the lower lashes. Excess shadow falls onto the tissue, not your skin.

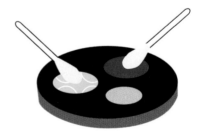

✳ Sweep taupe shadow in the crease to create natural-looking depth to the eyes.

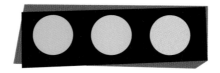

✳ If you have crepey eyelids, stay away from any type of shimmering shadows. Stick with sheer, silky, matte neutrals.

✳ Sweep powder shadow over eyeliner to soften the line.

✳ Gone overboard? Sweep a little translucent loose powder over your eye shadow to soften the color.

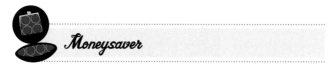

Moneysaver

Crush-n-play! If you break a powdered shadow, don't toss it. Put the pigment into an empty, clear, sealable container and crush it into a loose shadow; you can use up every pretty bit.

* If your lids have become veiny or discolored, apply a little foundation or an eye shadow primer to create an even lid before applying shadow. Colors stay truer longer, too.

* If you wear glasses, go easy on the eye makeup; your frames already draw attention to your lovely peepers. Stick with soft, neutral eye shadow shades and finish your look with a thin eyeliner line and mascara only on your upper lashes.

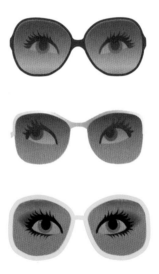

* If you wear contact lenses, apply your eye makeup first and then put in your contacts.

The Nasties

NOT—SO—PERKY PEEPERS

Try French blue eye drops to get the red out of tired eyes. The blue color makes the whites look whiter. You can find these in boutique pharmacies or online.

Keep a supply of water—soaked black tea bags in your freezer. Apply two of these icy compresses whenever your puffy eyes need a soothing cool—down.

Applying cold cucumber or kiwi slices can reduce puffiness. A spa treatment and snack in one!

"I keep two metal dessert spoons in the freezer. I place those babies against my eyes to chill out any puffies."

—ANNA, 25

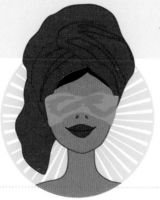

✳ Tend to see red? Stay away from pink-toned eye shadows that amplify redness in and around the eyes.

✳ If your eyelids are sensitive and become flaky when you wear eye shadows, you might be allergic to mica particles. Avoid shimmery powder shadows that contain glitter; they can irritate delicate skin. Instead, try an opalescent cream shadow.

✳ With colored eye shadows like blue or purple, concentrate on the lid area from the lash line to the crease. Don't color over the entire eye from lash line to brow bone unless you're singing "Send in the Clowns."

Budget Beauty

 TIPS FROM LADIES LIKE YOU!

"Vaseline as eye makeup remover! It takes everything off—including waterproof products—while moisturizing your eyelids. I gently rub Vaseline over my makeup and wipe away everything using a soft tissue."

—TRISHA, 18

Timesaver

Fast evening eyes: Sweep a glitter eye shadow across the lid from the lash line to the crease and smudge it under the lower lash line.

 Glamazon

For intense eye looks that last, first apply cream shadow. Then layer a matching shade of powder shadow on top.

✳ Avoid nasty cream shadow creasing. When wearing colored creams, dab shadow only on the lid. Use a powder shadow in the crease. This creates the subtle cream look without the fold-y crease.

✳ Young women can look great with sheer washes of bright cream shadow like teal or purple across their lids. Skip the eyeliner to keep it looking cool.

 Summer Beauty

Cream shadows can melt off your eyes or crease in summer's heat. For staying power, choose sheer washes of powder shadow.

✳ Super-oily skin can cause shadows to crease. Before applying shadow, try a dab of mattifying gel across the crease; it can help keep your color looking fresh.

✳ Instant eyelift! Use brightening concealer to draw a line from the outer tip of your brow to the outer edge of your eye and blend it for a beautiful finish.

✳ Wake up your eyes. Apply a little brightening concealer at the inner corners. This area tends to deepen and darken with age. A touch of light offsets the darkness.

✳ For a slick-n-sexy eye look, dab a little Vaseline over your eye shadow.

✳ Get festive for evening! Try some jewel-toned shadows. I love using an emerald shade on the top lid and smudging an amethyst shade along the lower lash line.

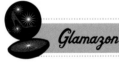 *Glamazon*

Go high-glam modern. Try pairing metallic eye shadows with neutral cheeks and lips. The best metallic shade for light skin is silver or platinum. Olive or medium skin tones look great with bronzes and golds. Darker skin looks fabulous with any metallic hue.

Tip Me, Carmindy

Q: *"How can I open up squinty-shaped eyes?"*

—FELICIA, 19

A: Sweep a highlight shimmer across the lid. Curl your lashes and coat them with black mascara for an eye-opening effect.

Q: *"I would love to wear eye shadow. But every type seems to accentuate my wrinkly eyelids. Am I missing a trick?"*

—DENISE, 48

A: Stay away from shimmery shadows; instead, experiment with sheer matte shades.

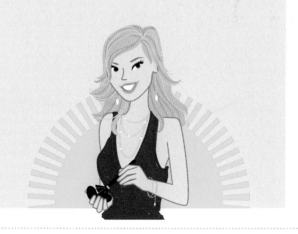

Q: "My eyes are so dark they look black if I'm not in direct sunlight. What should I do to liven them up—especially for a party?"

—JESSICA, 17

A: Play with shimmering, pale eye shadow shades. They'll be a great contrast to your gorgeous ebony eyes.

Q: "How can I achieve a smoky eye without looking like I lost a boxing match?"

—NATALIE, 30

A: Go easy on the shadow. Start with a light application, gradually building up the depth by blending every step of the way. Also try colors like quartz-y amethyst or sparkling brown instead of grays and blacks, for a lighter, more modern look.

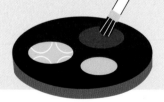

Seasonal Switcheroo

Spring/Summer

Take your beauty cues from the ultimate authority: Mother Nature. She changes things up; so should you!

Play with floral shades like roses and pinks; put away dark shades like wines and burgundies.

Sweep a little shimmery golden bronzer over self—tanned skin to accentuate your glow.

Pink lips look great on self—tanned faces. This combo also makes your teeth appear whiter.

A bright coral lipstick topped with a sheer, shimmery bronze gloss perks up your entire face, no matter what your skin tone.

For a relaxed and pretty daytime look, add a subtle wash of eyelid color (I like blue or green) and a dab of lip balm.

The Nasties

BIKINI LINE BUMPS

Before donning your swimsuit, apply a little spray foundation onto any unsightly red bumps that would be visible to your fellow beachcombers. Spray foundation covers well, plus it's a little water—resistant so it should stay put after a quick dip.

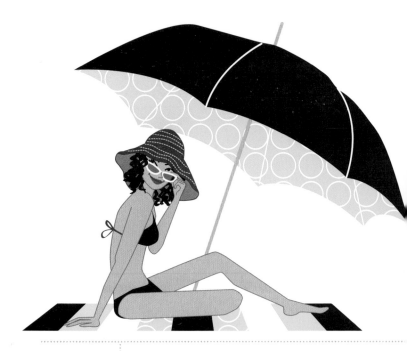

Two-in-one fun: Sweep bronzer onto your cheeks and across your eyelids for a fast sunny look.

Bewitching golden eyes: Apply a sweep of gold shadow across your eyelids and finish with black mascara on your lashes. Pale gold suits fair skin, tawny gold highlights medium skin, bronze—gold looks great on dark skin.

Summer loveliness: Apply bronzer to your temples, along the sides of your face, and under your cheekbones. Finish with a pop of bright pink blush on the apples of your cheeks and a slick of protective lip balm.

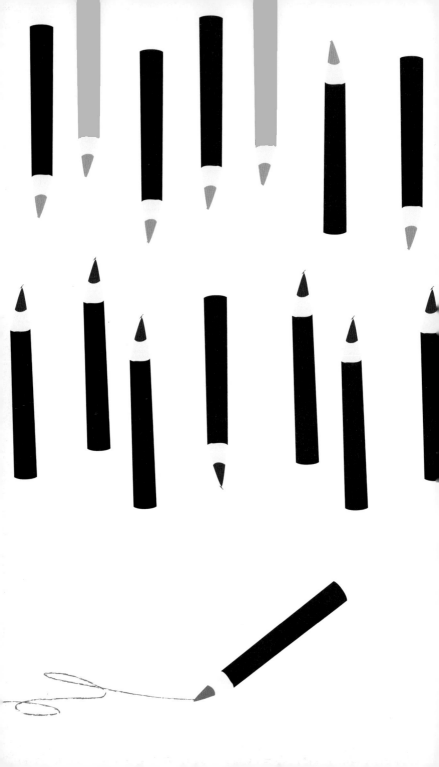

6

Eyeliner It Up

Lining the eyes is a surefire way to draw attention to your sultry stare. Cleopatra and her Egyptian pals (boys included!) got the kohl rolling. Nowadays we can quickly create a gorgeous glance using pencil, powder, liquid, or gel eyeliners. Play around and find what works best for you.

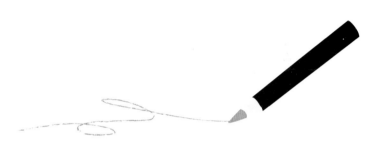

Always apply eyeliner before your mascara. If you try to line after mascara, you'll likely end up with a case of lashes clumps.

 * When applying eyeliner, start at the inside corners and work your way out. This encourages a natural-looking progression from thinnest line at the corners to thickest at the outside edges.

 * After lining, check for any gaps between your lash line and the eyeliner. If you're showing a bit of lid skin, fill it in with a few light strokes.

✳ Lining Physics 101: The thinner and sharper the pencil tip, the more precise the line. The fatter and duller the tip, the smudgier the line.

✳ Best pencil liner application technique ever: For upper lids, place that pencil at your inner eye corner. Look down into a hand mirror, and wiggle the pencil right into the lash line working your way outward.

✳ If your pencil liner needs sharpening, but seems too soft and keeps getting eaten by your sharpener, stick it in the freezer for a bit. This hardens the tip so you can sharpen it perfectly. Once it returns to room temperature, you're ready to start lining.

✳ Pencil liner gone all stubborn and difficult to apply? Try twisting the tip between your warm fingers to heat it up a little; it should draw on smoothly. Or blast the tip with your hair dryer for a second; the color will glide right on.

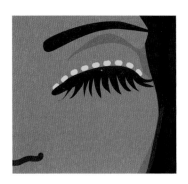

✳ Avoid perfection panic when applying pencil or liquid eyeliner. For better control, sweep it on in small strokes, like you're connecting little dashes.

✳ Create a thicker-looking, higher-impact lash line by wiggling your eyeliner under the roots of the upper lashes.

✳ Create a stencil for your liquid liner. Apply pencil liner first, then trace over that line with the liquid formula. Think of it as your path to a perfect line.

✳ Never use liquid liner under the lower lash line. It always looks too harsh.

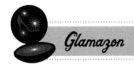

Glamazon

Extend your eyeliner just past the outer corner of the top lid, as if you were creating a last eyelash. This elongates your eyes and punches up the drama.

✳ Using a free finger, pull your temple back a little when creating a precise winged eyeliner look. Tautly pulled skin makes for an easier canvas.

✳ To hide the seam of false lashes, paint over it with black liquid liner.

✳ Dip an angle brush into powder eye shadow and run it across the lash line for an easy, soft look.

✳ To up the intensity, dip an angle brush in a little liquid transformer, water, or Visine, and turn your powder eye shadow into a precise liquid liner that dries to a nice powdery finish.

✳ Gel eyeliner is easier to apply than liquid but offers a similar finish. Wet a thin eyeliner brush (like the ones that come with liquid liners) and drag it through the gel liner. Wait a beat so it's not super-wet, then stroke it along the upper lash line. Easy, dreamy!

✳ Gel eyeliner is creamier than other types. It also adds a touch of hydration to the lash line, making it a great choice for ladies with drier skin.

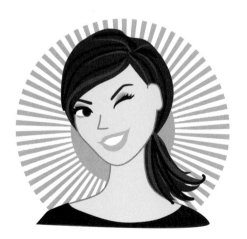

＊ To make eyes appear wider-set, start lining at the midway point and move outward.

＊ To make eyes appear closer-set, start lining at the inner corners and stop before you get to the outer edges.

＊ To deepen and intensify your natural eye color, take a black pencil and line the upper lash line on top of the roots. Then line the underside of the upper lash line with a pencil that matches your iris's shade.

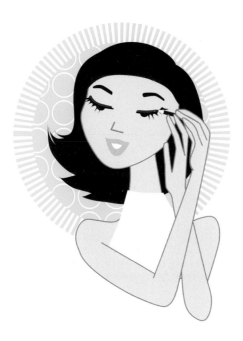

Opposites Attract

For eyes that pop, go for my "opposites attract" technique:

- To make *green eyes* really sparkle, apply a plum liner.
- For radiant *blue eyes*, use brown liner.
- To intensify *brown eyes*, try navy liner along the upper lash line.
- *Hazel eyes* look golden when you apply forest— or jade—green liner along the upper lash line.

A smudge of chocolate brown liner along the upper lash line—as close to the roots as possible—looks great on everyone.

* Teens should skip very dark black and gray liners: they look too harsh and heavy. Stick with natural browns for school and fun shades like purple, teal, blue, or metallics for weekends.

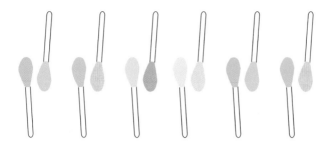

* Switch up your eyeliner shades as you age. Black tends to look a bit harsh. Opt instead for a soft slate or brown.

* Use a flesh-colored pencil on the inside rims of the eyes to intensify the whites of your eyes.

* Heavy, thick eyeliner ages mature faces. Line your eyes as close to the roots as possible.

* The softest way to line the lower lashes is to smudge a little eye shadow underneath them using an angle brush.

* For liner that won't budge or smudge, apply liquid liner. Then, using an angle brush, top it with a sweep of powder shadow in the same shade. This softens the look as well.

* To create doe eyes, dip an angle brush into a little powder shadow and sweep it on the outer top half of your upper lash line. Next, smudge a little shadow under the lower lash line, from the middle toward the outer corners. This opens up the eyes for that wide-eyed innocent look.

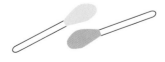

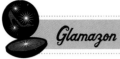

Glamazon

For a super-sexy rock-n-roll look, apply black liner on the top and bottom inside rims of the eyes, and then shut them really tight. OK, guitar goddess, now open your eyes. Using an angle brush dipped into a little black powder shadow, smudge the top and bottom lash line, staying very close to the roots.

To achieve a perfect winged-out cat eye with liquid liner, take a small-tipped concealer brush dipped into a little foundation and clean up around the wing. This corrects any unevenness, creating perfect edges every time.

Glamazon

For a modern metallic look, try double-stacking your liner. Line the upper lash line with a dark shade like black or brown, then apply a bronze or gold shade right over the top of that. Hot!

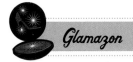
Glamazon

Apply a small dash of silver or gold eyeliner right on the center of your upper lid on top of your regular eyeliner for a flash of nighttime sparkle.

✳ For a wide-awake look, use cobalt-blue liner on the lower, inner rims of the eyes.

✳ If your eyes are small, keep your eyeliner line as thin and close to the roots as possible.

✳ With petite peepers, avoid rimming the insides of the eyes. One exception: use white or other light-colored pencils on the inside rim to brighten the eyes. That works wonders on everyone.

✳ If your eyes are large, feel free to draw on a thicker line of eyeliner.

✳ If you have deep-set eyes, steer clear of heavy black eyeliner. Choose lighter colors like brown or green to bring out those bedroom eyes.

✳ If your lids are a bit heavy and get smudgy easily, use waterproof liquid or pencil liner. Apply it while looking down, and then wait a beat for the liner to set and dry before looking back up.

* Asian eyes look incredible with just a chic slick of black waterproof liquid liner along the upper lash line.

* Wear contacts? Avoid lining the inner rims of your eyes. Eyeliner can travel underneath your lenses, causing irritation and redness.

* If you're prone to dark under-eye circles, skip lining the lower lash line.

* Place a dot of pearlescent white pencil on the inner corners of the eyes for a fresh, awake appearance.

* In a pinch, mascara can pull double-duty as eyeliner. Use an angle brush to pick up a little color from the mascara wand and smudge it into the lash line.

* For a funky night out, try liners that contain shimmer. You'll reflect every beam off that disco ball!

Summer Beauty

Waterproof eyeliners in fun colors like blue or teal look great during the summer. Plus they won't slip off in humid weather.

✳ For a smudgy, sexy look, rub some black eyeliner pencil onto your ring finger and mix a little dab of lip balm or Vaseline into it. Lightly smudge this concoction along the upper lash line using a Q-tip.

Glamazon

For a fun sixties retro look, apply black liquid liner along the upper lash line and slightly wing it out into a cat's eye. Next, draw a white pencil liner just under the wing at the outer corners.

✳ Kick up your party look! Line the upper lash line with one fun shade like teal. Then smudge the lower lashes with a different color like amethyst. Keep the rest of your makeup neutral.

✳ For smoldering eyes, line the lash line with a dark pencil—like jade, navy, or black. Smudge another color in the same family, but one or two shades lighter, next to the darker liner.

✳ If you have sensitive eyes, stay away from eyeliners that contain shimmery mica. Mica crystals can scratch delicate tissues and cause irritation.

 Timesaver

Save blending time and cash. Buy eyeliners that have built-in smudging tips on the other end. You won't need an angle brush or extra Q-tips.

✳ Have shaky hands? Stay away from liquid liners. Instead, pick up an angle brush and try powder liners. They're easier to manage and cleanups are a breeze.

 Timesaver

In a major rush? Smear a bit of pencil liner at the outer corners of the upper lash line. Run your finger over it to blend in a flash.

✳ If your eyeliner looks a tad too dark, sweep some face powder over it with an angle brush to soften the shade.

✳ If your eyeliner tends to run, switch to waterproof pencils. They stay in place all day long.

✳ If you've lost a few eyelashes, dot on a fine point of black pencil eyeliner to fill in the gap.

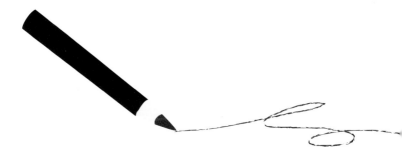

✳ Ladies, if your eyesight is not so great, don't guess where you're putting your liner. Get a major magnifying mirror—10x or 15x magnification—to get in there and see what you're doing.

Tip Me, Carmindy

Q: *"With age, my eyes have taken a downturn. My liner now points down at the outer edges no matter how I try to wing it. Should I just stop using liner?"*

—ESTHER, 59

A: *You can still use liner but skip the winging. Instead, stop the liner at the end of your eyes. Use a brightening concealer at the outer corners blending up to the end of your brows;*

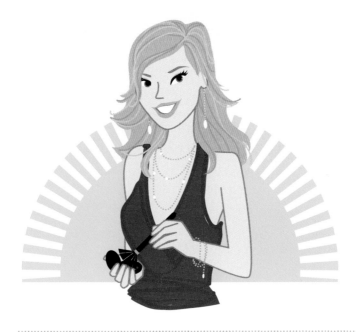

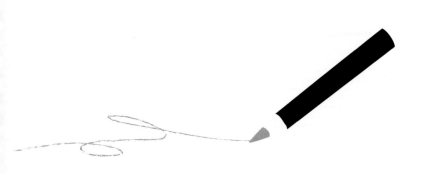

this lifts the eye. Curling the outer corner lashes and applying an extra coat of black mascara at the outer corners can also help bring up the eyes.

Q.: "If my eyeliner on one eye is too heavy, is there an easy way to even things out without starting from scratch?"

—SERENA, 29

A.: Sure. Take a small-tipped concealer brush dipped into a little foundation. Trace over the heavier part of the liner to erase the excess until you've got it all evened up.

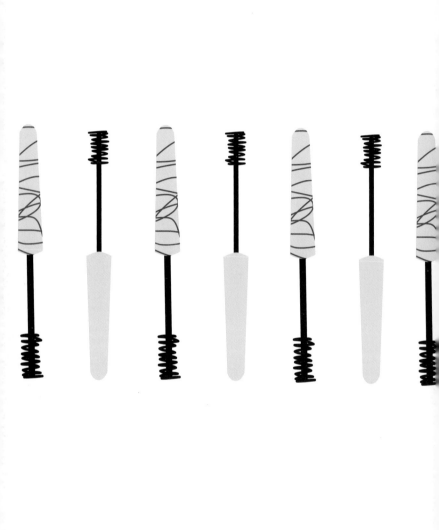

7

Luscious
Lashes

We all covet a fabulous black fringe of full-on lashes! It seems so unfair that the lushest ones are always gifted to babies and guys. We paint, coat, curl, and glue ours to create a look that opens doors with one little flirty batting. These lash tips aren't miracle-makers, but if you follow them, your eyelashes will look their very best. Lash out, lovelies!

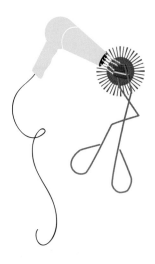

Straight-lash ladies, always curl your lashes to open up the eyes. Start at the base and squeeze for a few seconds. Work your way up, repeating the steps until you've curled the tips.

✳ For extra curling oomph, lightly run a warm hair dryer over your lash curler for about thirty seconds before crimping your lashes. Touch it with a clean finger before proceeding. You want it warmed, not scalding. Protect that delicate skin!

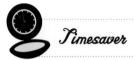

Timesaver

Overslept? Curl your outer lashes for a lightning-speed lift to your sleepy peepers.

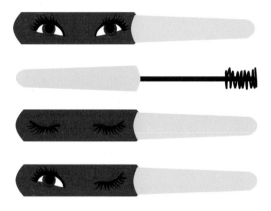

* Try the new smaller lash curlers. A mini-curler has a tiny clamp that grabs small sections of lashes, offering more precision and better control. You'll be less likely to pull out lashes or pinch the lids than with full-lash curlers.

* Mascara is one of my "must have on a desert island" products. Intensifying your lash line is the quickest way to frame your gorgeous peepers with a flirty fringe of fabulosity. Just sweep and go. No matter what shape, color, or size your eyes are, mascara enhances their beauty.

✳ If you're going to curl your lashes, always do it before mascara, NEVER afterward. Mascara sticks to curlers and you'll end up yanking out lashes, not to mention yelling in pain.

✳ To create your own lash plumpers, apply mascara and, while your lashes are still wet, dust them with loose powder and then reapply more black mascara.

✳ For a more dramatic, thicker mascara look, hold the wand vertically and brush back and forth.

✳ Always apply mascara to the bottom lashes first, then the upper lashes. If you do the reverse, when you tilt your head down to apply the mascara to the lower lash line you will smudge all your handiwork on the upper lid.

✳ When applying mascara to the bottom lashes, coat the top sides of the lashes starting at the base and sweeping toward the tips. Always coat the underside of the upper lashes starting at the roots and wiggling the brush up toward the tips.

✳ Avoid clumps by wiping excess mascara off the wand before starting your application.

✳ To wipe off a mascara wand, don't use toilet paper. It leaves a fuzzy residue that can end up in your eyes. Instead, go for a lint-free paper towel.

 ✳ Don't pump the mascara wand in and out of the tube before applying. That action breaks down the brush bristles and pushes air into the tube—drying out your mascara faster.

 ✳ I prefer using black mascara on everyone. Black creates more impact with less product.

 ✳ Hair color offers a general guide for everyday mascara shade. Blondes, redheads, and gray-haired gals, go for brown mascara. Brunettes and raven-haired ladies should stick with black.

 ✳ The best way to separate clumps after applying mascara is with a folding metal lash comb, not a plastic one. Its teeth are finer and stiffer and get the job done.

 ✳ In a pinch, you can use a toothpick to separate clumps in your lashes. It is a bit dangerous, so make sure no one can barge in and startle you. Also not a good idea if you're living on a fault line. Your sight is more important than perfect lashes, OK? Note to Ms. Toothpick: Go get a metal lash comb today.

 ✳ Never try and separate lashes after they have dried. They'll revolt and bolt from your lash line, leaving you with bald spots.

✳ Attention party girls! To make a serious lash statement, go for large-brush volumizing mascaras—sweeping two coats on both top and bottom. Look out!

✳ Not a fan of eye shadow? Check out tinted mascaras. Look for dark hues of deep green, navy blue, teak brown, or rich plum. Skip lighter shades; they're more distracting than alluring.

✳ If you are worried about lashes going limp after curling, keep them sky-high by applying waterproof mascara right after you curl. This tougher mascara formula keeps them in place, but can be rough on your lashes. So don't use waterproof mascara as your only mascara.

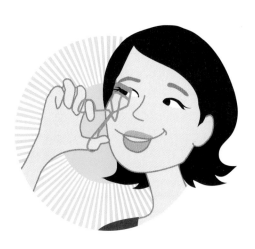

✳ If you have a wacky lash that bends in a crazy direction, avoid coating that one with mascara. Mascara will only enhance its wild streak. Keep it color-free so it fades into the background.

✳ To create well-separated lashes, twirl a clean, disposable mascara wand through them after your mascara. Buy them in bags of twenty-five at beauty supply stores. After use, quickly wash the wand clean of all mascara and let dry. You can reuse a single brush for a week before tossing it.

✳ For a natural daytime look, choose mascaras with small wands for precision and a light touch.

✳ To really open your eyes, apply a regular coat of mascara and let it dry. Then apply a second coat only to the outer corner lashes, both top and bottom.

✳ For a wide-eyed stare, apply mascara only along the outer half of the upper and lower lashes.

✳ If you're after a fast freshness, apply one coat of black mascara to only the top lashes. Mascara on the bottom lashes can mix with facial oil and run on you as you're running out the door.

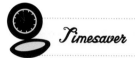

If you're in a real rush, simply sweep mascara across the very tips of your lashes. Flash-enhancement!

✳ Dried-out, crusty mascara can be liquefied by running the sealed tube under hot water for five minutes.

✳ Please heed the three-month replacement rule on mascara. Swollen, infected eyes are not hot.

✳ Eyelash curlers need maintenance, too. Always keep 'em clean. Replace the rubber pad every six months to ensure fabulous curl.

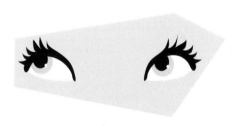

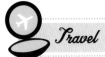

Travel

﹡ Have a salon professional tint your lashes before a beach vacation. You'll emerge from the waters looking like a mermaid and won't need to tote waterproof mascara.

﹡ When it comes to mascara, a bigger brush is *not* better. Larger brushes pick up more product, leading to more messy clumps.

﹡ Sometimes mascara misses the blondish lash roots. Touch up your roots with black liquid eyeliner.

Glamazon

For super-glam lashes, dust them with a little loose black-gold glitter while they are still wet with mascara. The glitter adheres better. When the light hits your lashes . . . Disco Diva!

﹡ If you want your lash line to look thicker, smudge eyeliner along the roots. This intensifies the line for a denser, fuller look.

﹡ False lashes are a flirty way to play up your eyes. Buy an inexpensive set at the local drugstore. Go for the most

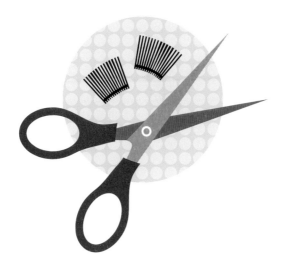

natural-looking ones you can find—not too thick or too long. Next, snip the falsies in half with scissors. Using lash glue, apply only these halves to the outside corners of the eyes. Going halfsies is easier to manage and looks fresher.

　❊ To fill in lash-line gaps, simply glue in a few individual false lashes to create a perfect fringe.

　❊ If you want a full set of false lashes, first hold them up to your eyes and check the length. They may need to be trimmed a bit to match your upper lash line. Snip off the excess, and then apply. For easier going, cut the whole set in thirds and apply one section at a time.

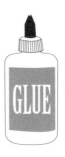

✳ When applying glue to a false lash, never squeeze the glue directly onto the lash band or your own lash line. Instead, squeeze out a drop on the back of your hand or on the container the lashes came in. Wait a few seconds for the glue to get slightly tacky. Drag the lash band through the glue so that a thin line of glue sits on the band. Now you're ready to stick it!

✳ I like using my fingers to apply small sections or full sets of false lashes. I use tweezers to drop in individual ones. They end up exactly where they need to be.

✳ Always apply false lashes first and then coat all your lashes with black mascara. This way the falsies will blend in perfectly with your realsies.

✳ Before applying false lashes, always curl your own lashes first with an eyelash curler so they blend with curled falsies. Never curl after putting on false lashes: you run the risk of pulling the false lash off and having to start over.

✳ If, after applying a set of false lashes, you have a visible seam, sweep liquid eyeliner along the lash line extending out just a bit at the corners. This blends the falsies into your lash line so no one will be the wiser.

✳ If you want longer-wearing falsies, head to a salon that offers semipermanent lash extensions. These are applied in sections with stronger glue to allow for about two to three weeks of flawless fringe.

Wacky Rituals

"I like to use regular mascara on the top lashes, waterproof on the bottom."

—HANNAH, 16

"Here's a lash-growing tip from my ophthalmologist. Every night after removing your makeup, lightly rub the rim of your eyelashes (top and bottom) with a damp cotton pad. Makeup tends to build up oils that clog the hair follicles and prevent growth. It may take a few weeks, but I swear my lashes are thicker and don't fall out so easily!"

—HELEN, 59

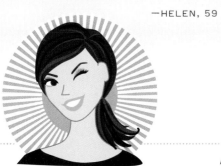

✳ For super-shimmery lashes, coat them first with black mascara. Once dry, paint shimmery gold or silver liquid eyeliner on a few lashes.

✳ If you don't like dark mascara but love lifted lashes, use an eyelash curler followed by a coat of clear mascara to hold the curl.

✳ Hold a plastic spoon behind your lashes when applying mascara. Any smudges wind up on the plastic, not your skin.

Glamazon

For a flirtatious look, apply mascara, then place a few individual false lashes only at the outer corners. Put a bit of glue on the back of your hand and lightly dip the small, knotted end into it. Wait a moment for the glue to become slightly tacky and then drop the lash into the outer edge of your lash line. Fun and kicky!

✳ Try sheer lash-tint mascara for a barely-there-but-lovely natural look.

✳ Got shaky hands? Purchase a tiny fan brush from the art supply store. Simply pull out the original mascara wand and sweep the tiny fan brush across it to pick up the color. Then lightly sweep it onto your lashes.

❋ Make the whites of your eyes look even whiter with this little trick. Apply cobalt-blue mascara to the baseline roots of your lower and upper lashes. Then coat the rest with black mascara. It works and is subtler than going with totally blue lashes.

❋ For light and easy lashes, apply one coat of mascara starting at the roots, wiggling the wand back and forth as you sweep up to the tips. Perfection!

❋ If you have alopecia, have undergone chemotherapy, or for other reasons are without lashes, eyeliner and shadow can work like magic. Line the upper lash line with a pencil. Then use an angle brush dipped into a matching shade of

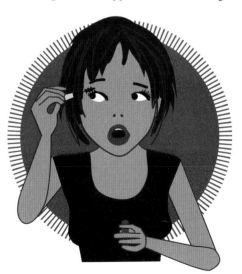

eye shadow to smudge shadow right over the liner. This creates a thick-looking lash line even if you're lash-free.

* Thickening mascaras build up lashes to create a denser look and are best for women with sparse lashes. The wands are compact and filled with bristles to grab lots of mascara. This ensures a gap-free, lusher look.

* Lengthening mascaras are best for women with shorter, stubbier lashes. Fibers in the formula adhere to your lashes and sweep out at the tips, giving the lashes a longer look.

* If you have trouble with mascara smudging, use the new tube-technology mascaras. These polymer formulas create little tubes around your lashes for a smudge-free, long-wearing lash. It's a breeze to remove; the tubes slip off with just a little warm water.

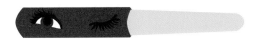

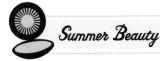

Summer Beauty

Tube-technology mascaras are especially great for women who find that their mascara runs by the end of a busy day, or live in hot, humid climates.

✳ Mature women should avoid waterproof mascara: it can cause brittle lashes. Opt instead for tube-technology mascaras, which coat your lashes without damaging them.

✳ Waterproof mascara should be worn only when swimming or in heavy humidity. Using it year-round can dry out your lashes and cause breakage. If you are a die-hard waterproof fanatic, try to at least alternate with a tube mascara a few days a week. Your lashes will thank you.

Winter Beauty

Avoid waterproof mascara during the cold winter months. Opt instead for protein-rich formulas that condition your lashes. They can really take a beating this time of year, so treat them gently.

✳ Lash primer helps create fatter lashes. Often white, this acrylic formula (which sometimes comes on the other end of a mascara) coats the lashes to give them extra girth. Follow with enough black mascara to cover all the white primer. This double-layer technique really beefs up scrawny lashes.

✳ Never apply mascara while driving a car, riding a jolty train, or any other situation where an accident could cause blindness. Duh!

✳ If you are prone to sties, pink eye, or other inflammation, you may want to invest in a bag of disposable mascara wands and use a new one each time you apply your mascara. This keeps bacteria away from your delicate tissues.

✳ If you have really sensitive eyes and find that mascara makes you itchy, try the all-natural hypoallergenic formulas found at most health food stores.

✳ Dab on a little leave-in hair conditioner to the top part of your lashes from time to time. It will keep them soft and supple.

✳ Take it easy when removing eye makeup, so as to not cause lash breakage. Never rub your eyes hard, either. Be nice to your little hairy friends: they keep you pretty!

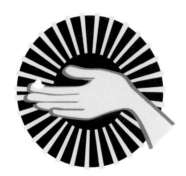

Tip Me, Carmindy

Q.: *"Mascara irritates my contacts. I end up teary and smudgy. My hairdresser says dying my lashes is a waste of time. Thoughts?"*

—ANNE, 52

A.: If your lashes are light, it is definitely not a waste of time to dye them. They will look darker and more defined. Also consider trying tube-technology mascara; it won't smudge or irritate your lenses.

Q.: *"I have very short lower lashes and can't really put mascara on them . . ."*

—STEPHANIE, 20

A.: Smudge a little powder eye shadow along the lower lash line using an angle brush. This creates the illusion of thicker, darker lashes without mascara.

Q.: *"Will applying clear mascara over black mascara create more definition?"*

—STACY, 24

A: No, but it can make the lashes look a bit shinier. If you curl your lashes, adding a top coat of clear mascara will also help hold that curl longer.

Q: "What if you blink or sneeze before your mascara is dry and you get those little black dots?"

—RENEE, 44

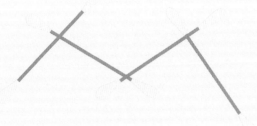

A: We have all done this and it's so annoying! Skip trying to clean it up with a Q-tip: it just reddens the area. Instead, grab a small-tipped concealer brush, dip it into a little foundation, and lightly brush away the dots. Perfection!

Q: "My long lashes have a tendency to smudge the brow bone, making a black mark there. How can I prevent this?"

—KATHLEEN, 62

A: Try tube-technology mascara or a waterproof formula: they don't budge. Make sure you keep looking down after you have applied any mascara and give yourself plenty of drying time before looking up. Maybe use the moment as your daily mascara meditation—a time to think of three wonderful things to look forward to that day.

Q: "Why do I always open my mouth when applying mascara? It's bizarre!"

—JOY, 40

A: Good question. My theory? We feel that stretching our whole face will allow the eyes and lashes to stand out so we won't get mascara on our skin. You probably also do it when you're trying to get something out of your eye.

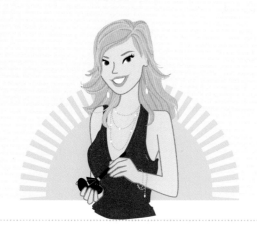

Seasonal Switcheroo

Fall / Winter

See the cooling change of seasons as an opportunity to break out of your makeup ruts and have some fun!

Play with deeper lip colors like sheer plums, rich berries, burgundy wines, and classic reds.

Warm up dull winter skin by mixing in a bit of cream bronzer with your foundation.

Wake up with a just—back—from—Bermuda glow by adding a drop of self—tanner to your nighttime moisturizer.

Eyeliner looks especially great with fall and winter fashions. Expand your liner lineup with enchanting shades like eggplant or chocolate brown. Pair your lined eyes with a nude lip for a chic, sophisticated look.

For family gatherings like Thanksgiving, keep your makeup simple and classic. Try a wine—stained lip paired with a soft brown shadow on the eyes for a universally flattering look Grandma will love.

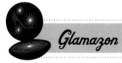

Glamazon

Glam up your office holiday party look while staying polished and professional. Add just a touch of glitter right at the center of your eyelid, very close to the lash line, over the top of your eyeliner. You'll sparkle, but not startle.

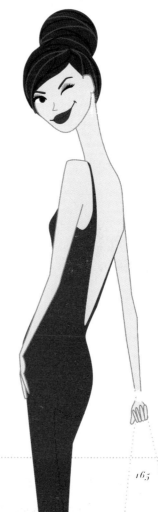

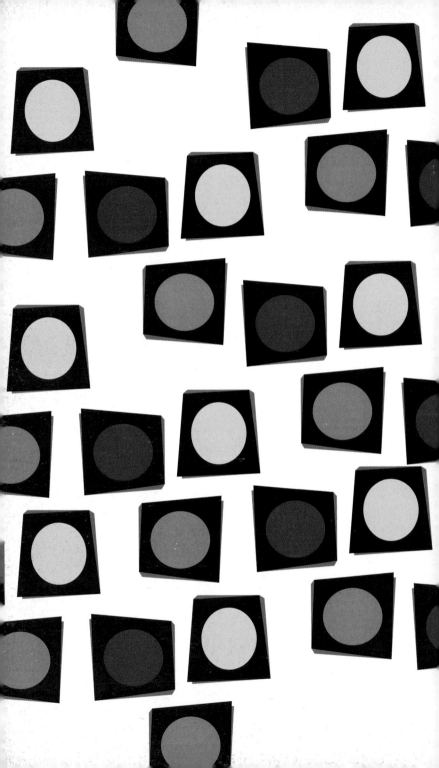

Get Cheeky

Whether you're eighteen or eighty-eight, a dab of blush wakes up a face like nothing else. Blush mimics youthful vitality. Playing up your cheeks can keep you looking "in the pink" even when you're feeling plowed under! We all know that looking fresh has a funny way of putting new pep in our step. When you need a lift, skip the coffee and grab that blush brush, beauty!

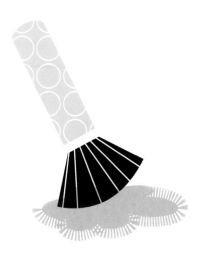

* Light skin looks loveliest with blushes in the peach or pink family.

* Ladies with medium-toned skin, play up your cheeks with mauve, rose, or terra-cotta blush shades.

* For gals with chocolaty skin tones, the brighter the blush shade the better.

* Dark-skinned ladies should avoid dull, brown blush colors: they look muddy. Instead, choose bright bold floral shades and blend on lightly for a fresh look.

* Rose blushes provide a natural, youthful flush for mature women.

* Blushes from the coral color family are universally flattering. When in doubt, go coral.

✳ Never change your blush color just to match your outfit or lipstick. Blush should always look like a natural pretty flush, not an accessory.

✳ Apply blush almost at the end of your full makeup application. Chances are you will see you only need a light sheer sweep of color to bring life to your cheeks.

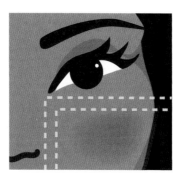

✳ Use the two-finger rule to find the best place to apply blush. Lay your index and middle finger side by side vertically next to your nose. You want to leave that much skin free of blush when approaching the nose. Place the same fingers horizontally under your eye. Keep that area clear as well.

✳ The easiest place to apply blush is on the apples of your cheeks. To find the apples, smile big; the prominent, round area is the apple.

✳ It's always best to use natural light whenever possible when applying blush. If it's too dark in the room, you run the risk of walking outside looking like a cartoon. Always check yourself in a few different lights before leaving the house.

✳ Whether applying cream, gel, or powder blush, always brush in upward strokes as to not drag down the skin.

✳ Keep powder blush from streaking or fading by prepping the skin with light foundation and powder first. This creates the perfect canvas for a soft cherubic flush that stays true.

✳ Use a big, fluffy powder brush to apply powder blush, not a regular blush brush. You'll achieve a much more diffuse, natural look and avoid the war-paint taint.

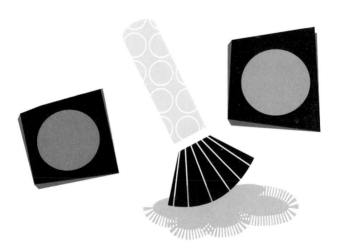

✳ Never use the blush brush that comes in the compact. It's too small and delivers too much product in a small area. You end up with uneven application and need more blending time.

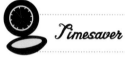

Timesaver

Powder blushes are a bit faster to apply than creams, because you don't have to blend as much.

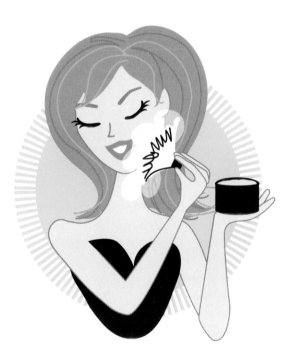

✳ Oily-skinned gals should stick to powder blush to create a smooth finish.

✳ Apply a bit of powder blush to the temples as well as the cheeks for a balanced, polished look.

✳ To apply a supersoft flush of powder blush, first dip your brush in loose translucent face powder and then into the blush color.

✳ To tone down overly applied powder blush, use a powder brush that has been dipped into a bit of loose translucent powder to dust over the blush—softening its impact.

✳ Ladies with really dry skin should opt for cream blush for a soft, moisture-enhancing finish.

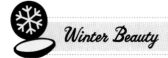

Winter Beauty

Normal-skinned gals should consider switching from powder blush to cream blush in the wintertime. As temperatures drop, your skin needs all the moisture it can get.

✳ Cream blush is the best option for mature skin: it restores radiance.

✳ To mimic a natural flush, swirl a dab of cream blush on the cheeks with your ring finger, using circular motions.

✳ Use a non-latex sponge to quickly, smoothly swirl on creamy blush. Flip it over to the clean side to buff the blush to a perfect finish.

✳ To lift an over-sixty face, apply blush toward the tops of the cheekbones for a healthy glow.

✳ If you're creating a dramatic night-time look with cream blush, try using a flat-top circular brush to swirl on color along the cheekbones.

✳ If you go a little overboard with your cream blush, there's no need to start over. Dip a makeup sponge in a bit of foundation and buff the cheeks gently to bring down the intensity.

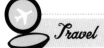

Travel

No blush? Use a dab of lipstick or colored gloss on the apples of the cheeks.

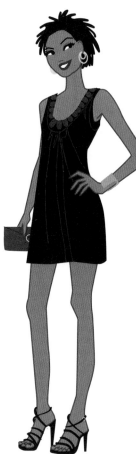

✳ If you find that cream blush streaks or disappears during the day, lightly dust a thin application of translucent powder on top to set it in place.

Moneysaver

Cream blush a shade too bright? Don't toss it. Mix in some tinted moisturizer to tone it down to a more wearable shade.

Glamazon

Here's the perfect no-fade blush technique for a wedding or other endurance test. First apply a natural cream blush. Sweep translucent powder on top. Add a pop of powder blush in a slightly brighter shade on top of that. You'll look peachy all day and night.

✳ Cheek stains offer a long-wearing blush. Cheek stains do not budge, look really natural, and are great for women who prefer a "no-makeup" look. Apply on the apples of the cheeks with a non-latex sponge and rub in circular motions. Work quickly, because stains dry in seconds and do not need to be set with powder.

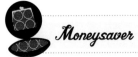

Moneysaver

Mix a drop of red food coloring and a bit of clear lip balm to make a quick and easy cream blush.

   * If you have mature skin, skip cheek stains. They can settle into fine lines.

   * If your skin is not very smooth, stick with soft matte blush formulas. Avoid shimmery blushes. Also skip cheek stains: they can settle into rough spots.

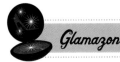

Glamazon

For drama, use two shades of cream blush. Swirl on a rosy hue to the apples of the cheeks then apply a lighter pink shade back along the cheekbones into the hairline for soft romantic definition.

   * Are you red-faced with can't-find-anything frustration? Time to streamline that makeup bag and drawer. Clear out that hoard of old samples, useless "gifts with purchase," not-quite-right shades, and that stuff from 1989. Ending clutter chaos feels great, and *that* looks good on you!

   * Cheeky checklist: remember that highlighter illuminates, bronzer deepens, and blush brightens.

* Just by applying cream highlighter to the tops of your cheekbones—and skipping the blush—you'll light up your cheeks and showcase the natural planes of your face.

* To highlight your cheekbones, take a fan brush and sweep powder highlighter onto the tops of the cheekbones in a C-formation. Start at the temples and sweep down along the tops of the cheeks.

* To give definition to the cheekbones, sweep a bit of bronzer under the hollows of the cheeks.

* To find the hollows of your cheeks, suck them in. The indented areas are the hollows.

 ## Glamazon

For hi-def glamour, sweep highlight on top of the cheekbones. Next, apply blush color on the apples and along the cheekbones back into the hairline. Finish with a sweep of bronzer under the hollows.

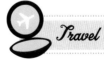 ## Travel

No highlighter? Blend a dab of clear lip gloss on the top of the cheekbones for a quick hit of glow-to-go.

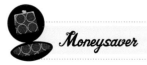

Moneysaver

Fridge fancy: press ice cubes on your cheeks for a fast, natural flush.

✳ Use a terra-cotta-colored blush or powder bronzer to mimic a lightly tanned cheek. Sweep it along the temples, sides of the face, and under the hollows of the cheeks.

✳ For an earthy, outdoorsy look, sweep a bit of bronzer only on the temples, cheeks, and across the bridge of the nose.

✳ Create a peachy cheek by applying highlight on the top part of the apples, a peachy pink on the apples, and a bit of bronzer right under the apples.

✳ Want sexy? Blend a bit of cream bronzer at the temples, into the hairline, and along cheekbones. Finish with a pop of bright color right on the apples.

Glamazon

Party girls, dust on a golden or pearlescent shimmer on top of your blush for extra pizzazz!

❋ To enhance round cheeks, blend a dab of highlighter on the top of the upper cheekbones. Finish with a swirl of colored blush right on the apples.

❋ To enhance flat cheeks, sweep highlighter in a C-formation from the temples, along the sides of the face, and then under the cheekbone. Sweep colored blush from the hairline across the cheekbones, stopping on the apples two finger-widths from the nose. Then suck in your cheeks and sweep a bronzer from the side of the face next to the ears down into the hollows.

❋ Glorify high cheekbones by smoothing highlighter along the tops and finishing with a shimmery blush.

❋ Define low cheekbones by sweeping a bit of blush a tad above the cheekbones instead of right on them.

❋ Compliment at least one stranger every week on her appearance. It's not cheeky; it's good karma! You have no idea the positive effect this will have on a woman, and it will make you feel good, too.

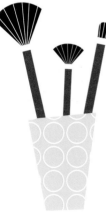

❋ Accentuate your dimples by blending a speck of bronzer in the indentation.

❋ When wearing bronzer, don't finish with much face powder: you'll look downright dusty.

✳ Older and wiser ladies, choose a sheer cream bronzer that contains no shimmer. It blends easily and won't settle into fine lines.

 ✳ To keep cream bronzer in place, very subtly apply loose translucent powder on top.

 ✳ Powder bronzer glides on smoothly if you first apply a light base of translucent powder.

Moneysaver

No bronzer? Mix a little shimmering brown eye shadow with a little loose face powder to sweep on some sun.

Winter Beauty

Avoid heavy bronzers during the cold winter months; it's not a natural look. Instead, opt for sheer washes of blush on the apples of the cheeks.

 ✳ For a really long-wearing blush look, try applying self-tanner only across the cheekbones. Most tanners last for about a week. Each morning, all you have to add is a pop of color on the apples.

✳ Best bet for a fast fresher-upper? A terra-cotta blush color swept on cheeks and lightly across your eyelids.

Timesaver

Dashing out in the evening? Kick up your morning blush with a second layer of shimmering blush. The more sparkling the shade, the more you'll glow in nighttime light.

✳ If you get a blush streak on the cheek, buff the entire area down with a clean non-latex sponge. Then subtly add back the amount of color you want. Don't correct a streak by filling it in with more color; that's a recipe for a rouge riot.

Travel

Stuck without any products? In a pinch, just pinch your cheeks like Grandma used to. This stimulates your skin's blood flow. You'll have a rosy smile in seconds!

Party Looks

Parties offer the perfect opportunity to play a slightly different role. Think: what image do I want to project tonight? Bohemian? Glamorous? Rock-n-roll? Preppy? Have fun creating a look that has a little extra pizzazz. It'll enhance your party mood. Who knows what might happen?!

Hollywood Glamour: Black liquid liner on the eyes, plus bold red lips.

Captivating: A sexy, smoky eye balanced with barely-there lip color.

Elegantly seductive: A ruby-stained lip with champagne-shimmer eyes.

Romantic: Try rose-colored lips and cheeks, with a soft brown shadow on the eyes.

Modern: Go for metallic accents of silver, gold, or bronze. But use these only on one feature at a time—eyes or lips or cheekbones.

California Beachy: Go for bronzed skin with a coral mouth.

Retro Sixties: Wear false lashes with black liquid eyeliner and a pale mouth.

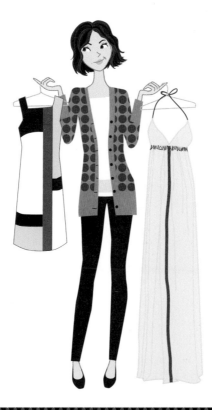

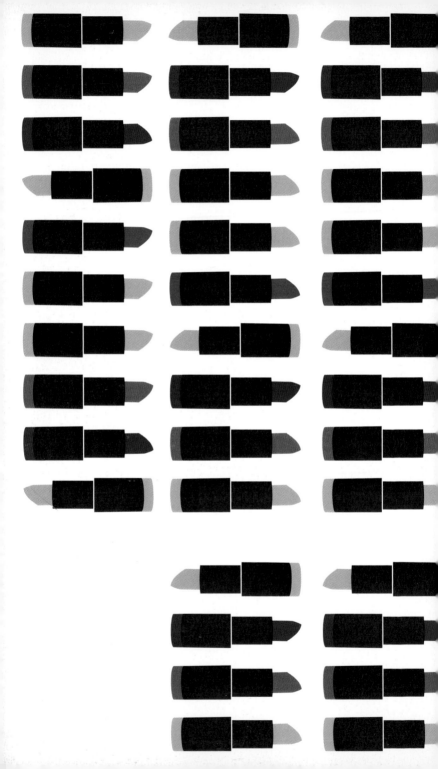

9

Lips, Lips, Lips

CrazyBusyBeautiful babes, lip color (or lippy, as my adorable Australian gal-pals call it) is your one-stop prettifying prop.

If you're feeling stressed out or tired, a bold or bright shade of lipstick can perk you up instantly. A new lippy is also the cheapest, quickest way to update your makeup wardrobe. Buy the hottest new shade to feel on top of your game.

Then use those luscious lips to speak your mind and heart. Sing it out, ladies!

＊ To get smooth lips, buff them with a toothbrush dipped in a little water and white sugar. Don't rub too hard. Always follow with a light balm.

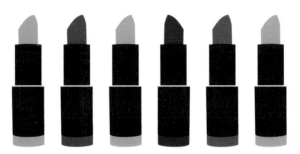

Best lip color shades for blondes: pinks, mocha pinks, peachy pinks, sandy pinks, cool corals, roses, mauves, berries, cherry reds.

Best lip color shades for brunettes: true pinks, roses, plums, bronzes, golden pinks, brownish pinks, shimmering mochas, coral, wines, true reds.

Best lip color shades for redheads: warm pinks, peaches, apricots, honey—colored nudes, sheer corals, raisins, gold—flecked reds.

Dark—skinned gals, go for these lip color shades: golds, honeys, caramels, oranges, deep corals, tangerines, deep plums, bronzy pinks, mahoganies, blackberries, maroons, blood reds.

Asian beauties, try these lip colors: sheer corals, pinks, roses, golden pinks, pinky browns, mauves, deep plum stains, shimmering beiges, nudes.

Ladies with mocha skin, head for these lip colors: sheer golds, beiges, coffees, caramels, toffees, bronzes, berries, plums, wines, true pinks, corals, sheer raisins, garnet reds.

If you're very fair—skinned, avoid super—dark lipstick. It's too harsh for you. If you like a deeper shade, go for the same hue in a gloss or a transparent lipstick.

Ebony beauties should avoid pastel lip shades. They can wash you out and look chalky.

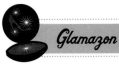
Glamazon

If you want to play with nude lip colors—à la Brigitte Bardot—make sure they contain a little hint of color. Otherwise you'll look sickly, not sizzling. For light skin, choose a peach or pink nudes; medium skin, choose tawny pink beiges; dark skin, go for caramels or mochas.

✳ The perfect daily lipstick is about two shades darker than your natural lip color. For most ladies, it's a rosy pink that enhances your natural shade by turning it up a notch.

✳ As we age, we should move away from heavy, dark, opaque lip shades. Opt for fresh, light neutrals or sheer rosy pinks that bring a youthful boost of color to the face.

✳ Don't pick your lip color according to your outfit. It's cheesy. Instead, go for shades that complement your skin tone.

✳ To make teeth look whiter, choose lip colors with a blue-based undertone. Stay away from warm or golden shades that have yellow-based undertones.

✳ To determine a shade's undertone, swipe the lip color onto white paper. Does it look more bluish or more yellowish? Voilà, you're a shade expert.

✳ Over-lining the lips never looks natural. There is no set standard of perfect lip shape! If you must use liner, don't ever use liners darker than your lipstick or gloss shade.

✳ If you must wear colored lip liner, trace the lip border with nude lip liner or one that matches your natural lip color. Lipstick will stay put without that severe ring-around-the-mouth look.

✳ Dab a little spot of highlight cream on those tiny shadows that can appear at the corners of the mouth. It bounces light from the area.

✳ Dump the plumper! Lip plumpers just irritate your lips, causing them to barely swell for a second. Learn to enhance your natural shape instead.

✳ Try lining the outside rim of your lips with a light highlighting pencil. It gives your pout a halo effect and makes lips look fuller. Or take a little highlighting cream or shadow and add a dab on top of the Cupid's bow of the lips and just below the lower lip. This also gives the illusion of naturally fuller lips.

* Pat just a little bit of shimmering lip gloss onto the center of the lower lip. By highlighting this one area, you give the lips the illusion of extra plumpness. By using just a touch, you avoid creating an overly slick look.

* Small lip tip: Avoid wearing dark lip colors; they make lips look smaller.

The Nasties

COLD SORES

Ugh. Cold sores are awful and awfully contagious. When treating and covering them, always use disposable Q—tips. After a swab touches the sore, toss it. Don't re—dip it in your product.

To hide a cold sore, first apply foundation everywhere *except* the infected area. Then use a Q—tip or a new, disposable sponge to dab foundation over the cold sore. Using a new swab or sponge, tap on a touch of yellow—toned concealer. Set it with a light dusting of powder using a new Q—tip.

＊ To create a prominent pout, do not draw on a big lip with lip liner. Instead, choose light or bright lip shades that contain shimmer. Shimmer catches the light for a magnifying effect.

＊ If your lips are large and you want color but not added fullness, choose shimmer-free neutral shades. Shimmer magnifies; a matte shade tones down volume.

＊ Daring and bold babes, choose a favorite strong lip color and make it your signature shade. Be legendary!

＊ Every woman can work a red lip. If you're fair, go for blue-based reds like strawberry or cherry red. Medium skin tones, try true reds like apple or fire-engine red. Dark skin looks amazing with blood reds and garnets. Redheads, you can play the red game with warmer shades like tomato and brick red.

＊ For long-wearing red lips, trace the perimeter of your lips with a red pencil (one of the very few times I recommend colored lip liner). Then use the liner to fill in the lips completely. Finish with red lipstick on top.

＊ When wearing bright or bold shades of lipstick, minimize makeup elsewhere on your face. Skip the clown appearance; create a balanced look.

✳ To keep your painted lips looking flawless, trace around the edges with a small-tipped concealer brush that has been dipped in a little foundation.

✳ If you wear red lipstick, skip the gloss topper. It's too messy and looks overdone.

✳ Want a pop of red without the full commitment? Try a sheer red gloss.

✳ Tinted lip balms are the most natural way to wear color while moisturizing and protecting your pucker-parts.

✳ Never lick your lips before applying lip color. It prevents the hue from sticking to your kisser.

✳ If your lips get chapped easily, don't wear flavored lip products. They encourage licking, which creates more chapping.

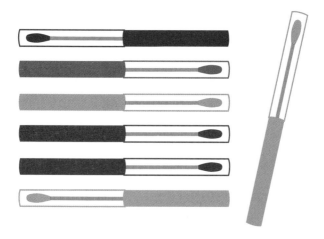

＊ Love gloss but have trouble keeping it on? Try applying a thin veil of matching colored lipstick first. Blot gently with a tissue. Next, swipe on the gloss. If it comes off, you're still working that leftover color underneath.

＊ To keep gloss from traveling across lip lines, line your lips first with a totally clear lip pencil.

＊ Lip stains provide a natural-looking tint, but they can be drying. After the stain dries, top your lips with a hint of clear gloss or balm.

＊ Only use lip stains when your lips are perfectly smooth; otherwise stains seep into the cracks. If you have lines around the mouth, skip lip stains, as they tend to bleed into the lines.

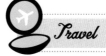

Travel

Blend a little cream blush onto your lips if you don't have your lipstick handy.

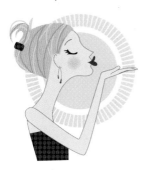

The Nasties

HICKIES

If a hot date has left you looking like Dracula dined on your neck, it's time to cool things down. Wet a metal spoon and stick it in the freezer. Once it's icy cold, take it out and hold it against your sucked skin.

A hickie is actually a little pool of blood under the skin. To fade a hickie faster, roll a closed lipstick tube over the area. This helps break up the blood so it disperses more quickly.

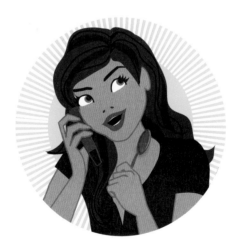

✳ The most natural way to apply lipstick is lightly from the tube. Be sure to run your finger over the top of your lips to soften the edges.

✳ But . . . applying lipstick with a brush makes it last longer. Going straight from the tube uses up more product.

✳ Use a lip brush for a perfectly painted-on lip. It takes a second longer to use a brush, but the finish is five times better.

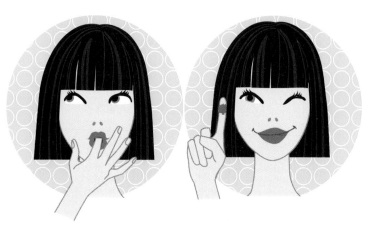

✳ To prevent getting lipstick on your teeth, stick your index finger in your mouth after you apply the lipstick. Purse your lips, and then pull out your finger. Excess lipstick winds up on your finger, not on your teeth.

✳ Mom was right. Blotting lipsticked lips with a tissue then reapplying makes lipstick last longer. Blotting removes oils in the lipstick—turning it into more of a lip stain. Adding the extra layer restores the color and moisture.

 ✳ Want to make lipstick last all night? Double up! Apply a lip stain, then your lipstick. Avoid gloss; it can speed color slippage.

 Summer Beauty

Don't slather on a load of lipstick in the spring and summer; if it looks thick, it looks wrong. Get a blossom-fresh look by first putting bright lip color on your finger. Press it into the lips for a stained, natural finish.

 ✳ For a party smile with extra punch, apply a clear gloss that contains glitter over your lipstick.

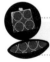 *Moneysaver*

Use every bit of your favorite lippies. Scoop out whittled down lipsticks and put each shade in a compartment of a little plastic pillbox for a great palette to mix and match.

Budget Beauty

TIPS FROM LADIES LIKE YOU!

"I think tinted ChapStick is better and cheaper than lipstick. Plus it comes in bonus-size packages."

—STACIA, 24

"When my gloss runs low, I cut the tube in half and use a lip brush to apply it on my lips. I use it all up before replacing it. To reduce the mess, I keep my gloss in an old film container, but any little plastic tub that seals would work."

—ERICA, 29

"Instead of strips, I whiten my teeth by dipping my tooth-brush in water or mouthwash and then a little baking soda. Brushing with this keeps stains at bay."

—LISA, 37

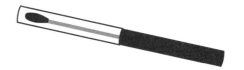

✳ Sudden change of lipstick heart? Don't just wipe off the lipstick with a clean tissue. Lingering color bits will mess with your new shade. Use a clean sponge dipped in a tiny bit of foundation to fully clear out the first color.

✳ To keep matte lipstick from looking dry and dated, apply a slick of balm first.

✳ Never apply lipstick at the table. So tacky! Either head for the ladies' room or try my sneaky lip trick. Under the table, pull out your lip color and apply it to your index finger. Then bring your finger up to your lips subtly and sweep it on.

✳ If you like opaque lipsticks, make sure they are creamy, moisture-infused formulas that won't dry out your lips.

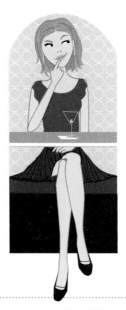

＊ Women over fifty should skip glossy or high-shimmer lipsticks. Stick with moisture-formula matte or semi-matte lipsticks for a polished look.

＊ Women under thirty can wear high-shine, super-gloss lipsticks for a party or night out. However, they're still a bit much for daytime.

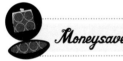

Moneysaver

Slicking on Vaseline is the original cheap-n-easy gloss. An oldie but a goodie!

＊ Create your own sheer lipstick by mixing an opaque lipstick with a hint of Vaseline.

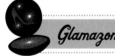

Glamazon

Mix loose glitter into a clear gloss or Vaseline for a serious party-girl look.

＊ For a berry, wine-stained look, apply wine-colored lipstick to your finger and then lightly tap it on your lips.

You'll look like you've been sipping merlot by the fire all night. Très sexy!

    ✳ A petite glam-slam: after applying gloss, add a dab of gold shimmer loose eye shadow on the center of the lower lip.

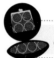 *Moneysaver*

Save money by playing Picasso. Instead of running out to buy new products, layer your lip colors to create new shades. Mix and match lipsticks, glosses, and all kinds of lip products together. Who knows what you might come up with in your loveliness laboratory!

    ✳ Heavy matte lipsticks are definitely passé. Embrace the new matte lipsticks that offer a creamy, sheer, moist finish.

    ✳ If there's a crazy new trendy color you want to buy, try a sheer gloss version first. You'll stay in fashion without looking like a fashion victim.

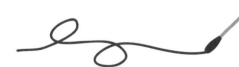

✳ If your lipstick color looks too dark or deep, brighten it by applying a much lighter gloss on top.

✳ If your lipstick looks too painted on, lightly trace a Q-tip around the perimeter to soften the edges.

✳ Some ladies' natural lips differ in color, with upper and lower lips being quite darker or lighter. For uniform lip color looks, first create an even canvas. Apply a light layer of foundation on the lips; follow with lipstick. Perfection!

Wacky Rituals

"I use whipped cream to soften my lips. It makes them feel fuller, healthier, and younger."

—CARMEN, 32

"For a sexy evening look, I dust a little shimmery eye shadow onto my lips before I apply lipstick. It truly makes the lipstick last much longer and also gives you an iridescent pout you just can't find in any tube!"

—COURTNEY, 23

"I stain my lips by dabbing on strawberry Jell-O powder. Tastes good, too!"

—MICHAELA, 26

✳ Lips that turn down at the corners create quirky cute smiles. Color for these lips looks best put mainly in the center, and then fading outward without reaching corners.

✳ To balance lips if the upper one is thinner and the bottom fuller (or vice versa), apply a slightly darker shade of lipstick on the larger half and a lighter shade in the same color family on the smaller half. Then blot those beauties together.

✳ Purse pointer: if you can carry only one product, it should be your lip color. Stash it with a retractable lip brush that twists to cover itself. No more lipstick smears all over your bag.

Timesaver

Fastest way to go from your work look to party-ready: simply sweep on a deeper or more shimmering lip color.

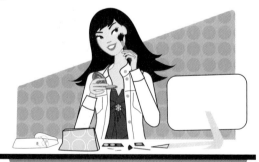

Summer Beauty

During the summer, be sure to use lip products with SPF. If your lip color doesn't offer SPF, apply a sunscreen lip balm before putting on your lippy.

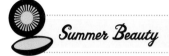 ## Winter Beauty

Double up on moisturizing during cold weather. Apply a moisturizing lipstick or gloss over lip balm to ensure chap-free, soft lips. Especially important under the mistletoe!

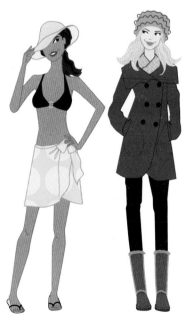

Tip Me, Carmindy

Q: *"Is there a lip shade that is flattering for women of all colors?"*

—DANIELLE, 33

A: *Rose lipsticks work on everybody. Redheads look great in warm rose; fair ladies shine in cool pink rose. Olive complexions win with true rose, and darker complexions beam with deeper rose. Also, don't be afraid of coral lip shades. They look great on everyone as long as they are sheer.*

Q: *"If you messed up the line of your pretty bow, how can you get your lipstick back to where it should be without making a smudge under your nose?"*

—ESTHER, 59

A: *Trace the upper lip line with a small-tipped concealer brush dipped in a little foundation to clean up the shape without smudges.*

Q: *"I had the worst chapped lips this winter. What's a good remedy to get my lips back into shape?"*

—ANDREA, 34

A: However tempting, don't pick at chapped lips. Instead, gently scrub them with a toothbrush dipped in Vaseline and white sugar. Rinse the flakes and sugar away; follow with a rich balm.

Q: "I had surgery and cannot wear eye makeup. What can I wear on the rest of my face so I still look polished?"

—ELIZABETH, 51

A: Play up your lips with a fab shade of lipstick to redirect the focus!

Q: "My lips are very wrinkly. What lipstick do I use so that they do not stand out or shimmer like tin foil?"

—BETHANY, 21

A: Go for a moisturizing matte lipstick; it will hide lines and make your lips look luscious.

Q: "Is lip gloss more casual and lipstick more formal, or does it matter when you wear them?"

—STEPHANIE, 20

A: A sheer gloss worn alone or lipstick in a neutral color worn alone can look casual, but for a more formal look I suggest wearing a rich lipstick with a slick of gloss on top.

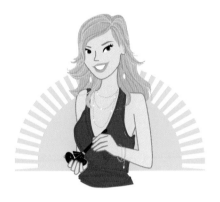

One Final Tip . . .

Believe in your unique beauty. Know you are lovely and lovable without a speck of makeup. At every age. Every day.

Don't you dare hide your light in the darkness of insecurities, comparison games, or other people's opinions. Go forth and conquer with confidence, girlfriend. Celebrate the glorious, gorgeous treasure that is YOU.

Be positively beautiful. Because that's what you are!

Love,

Carmindy

Acknowledgments

I would like to thank these brilliant people, each of whom never ceases to inspire and support me. They make life and work a fun and fabulous journey—proving that professional success and personal happiness can and should always go together. Kitchen Table Productions forever!

* Sarah Burningham—the true visionary behind this book. She dreamed it, shared it, and encouraged it. She shines that radiant light that is pure beauty.

* Joy Bergmann—a stunning example of genius, professionalism, and creativity. I simply can't live without her.

* Jay Sternberg—my touchstone, my heart, and my soul. Especially when I'm crazy, busy, and not feeling so beautiful!

∗ Gay Feldman—her encouragement and advice help me move mountains.

∗ Ashleigh Cucci—her can-do attitude and fantastic humor help get me through it all.

∗ Chrissy Lloyd—she not only dresses me beautifully, she has helped me see that art is everywhere.

∗ Peter Buckingham—photographer extraordinaire. He always nails it!

∗ Noah Hatton—his brilliance and honesty have blessed me for years and years.

∗ Myrdith Leon-McCormack—a bright, sunny gift on a cloudy day.

∗ Amy Saidens—she captures women's wonderfulness like no illustrator I know.

∗ Lacy Sakert—a fountain of fun ideas frequently served up poolside with cocktails.

∗ Sun Studios—these pros always greet me with smiling faces and good deals.

∗ Jack, Julie, and Quinn Bowyer—my family, whom I love more than words can express.

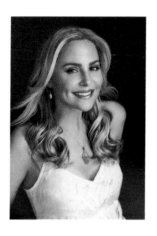

As the makeup artist on TLC's hit show *What Not to Wear*, Carmindy has redefined beauty for everyday women. She's the cocreator of a natural line of cosmetics called Sally Hansen Natural Beauty inspired by Carmindy, and the author of *The 5-Minute Face* and *Get Positively Beautiful*. Her work can also be seen in *Cosmopolitan; Elle; InStyle; O, The Oprah Magazine; Essence; Self; Lucky;* and *Marie Claire*. Read Carmindy's weekly blogs on www.dailymakeover.com or visit her at www.carmindy.com.

You are invited to try

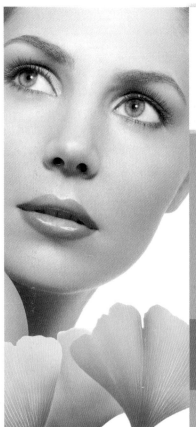

Sally Hansen®
natural Beauty™
inspired by CARMINDY

Finally, cosmetics that reveal your natural beauty

Revolutionary formulas infused with natural ingredients that care for your skin

PARABEN-FREE

Developed by Sally Hansen® with the expertise of Carmindy

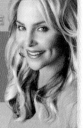

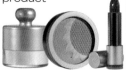
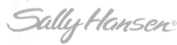